FACES OF
MENTAL ILLNESS

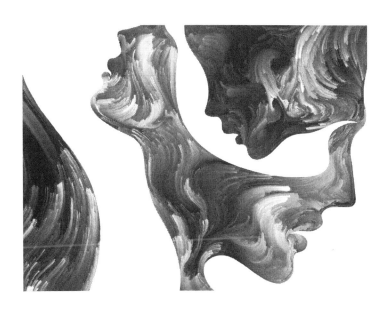

CLAUDIA FERNANDEZ-NIEDZIELSKI
SAMANTHA RUTH
KATE BUTLER

FACES OF
MENTAL ILLNESS

20 STORIES BRINGING YOU THROUGH
YOUR JOURNEY FROM STIGMA TO HEALTH

Foreword by Jack Canfield, co-author of
Chicken Soup for the Soul® series

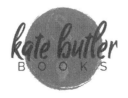

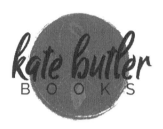

First Edition

www.katebutlerbooks.com

ISBN: 978-1-952725-20-3

Design by Melissa Williams Design
mwbookdesign.com

I dedicate this book to my parents, Isidoro and Marina,
to my younger brothers, Alex and Leo; to my aunts Concha,
Maria Elena, Laura and Gina;
to the entire Gerber Family, to the town of Lester, IA and the surrounding
community and to Dr. Martha Ontiveros and the staff at the
Instituto Nacional de Psiquiatria, Mexico City

You are all part of my history and my story.
Each one of you, in your own way, stood by me in my darkest moments
and were instrumental to my recovery.
I owe you my life and will be forever grateful.

To John, Christopher and Samantha, my husband and children,
I dedicate this book and my life to you.

You have given me more than I could have ever imagined as
I am fully aware that it has not been easy living with me.
Your love, understanding and kindness through my darkest moments
have meant more than I will ever be able to vocalize.
If I ever hurt you, neglected you, or ignored you during my mental cycles,
please forgive me, as I have never meant to cause you any pain.
You give meaning to my life and I will forever love you!

Claudia Fernandez-Niedzielski

To my family, thank you for loving and believing in me…
even when I didn't love and believe in myself.

To Kate Butler, thank you for being you,
for your unconditional love and support, and for
believing in us and this movement.

To Claudia, thank you for your passion,
your friendship and love,
and your commitment to changing the way the world views Mental Illness.

And to my late husband Jim, who I love with every fiber of my being,
thank you for seeing me, for accepting me, and
for loving me exactly as I am . . . WITH Anxiety and PTSD.

This wouldn't be happening without all of you in my life and
by my side every step of the way.
You make my world a better place just by being in it.

All of my love, Foreveralways.

Samantha Ruth

Together we dedicate this book to YOU.
To each and every person that holds this book, reads this book,
shares this book . . .
to all those who live with a mental illness and continue
to push forward every day;
to their families and loved ones, for their support, love and understanding;
and to all mental health service providers who continue to find ways to
improve our lives and find the best treatment for each one of us.

We want you to know that you're NOT alone.
We want you to know that what you perceive as your disadvantages
are actually your gifts. We want to give you hope.

Hope that you will get through this.
Hope that you will grow stronger through this journey.
Hope that the world will soon catch up and recognize
that stigmas only add to our struggles
and compassion and connection are what's missing.

We hope that you will hear the strength we've gathered
through using our voices.
We hope you recognize that silence is the enemy.
We hope you gain a glimmer of what
your life can and WILL be if you just keep going.

Please know we get it. We've been there. And we're here for you!

DISCLAIMER

This book contains the opinions and ideas of its authors. It is intended to provide helpful and informative material on the subjects addressed in the publication. It is sold with the understanding that the authors and publisher are not engaged in rendering medical health or any other kind of personal professional services in the book, and that the ideas expressed in this book are not to be taken as endorsements or recommendations for the reader to follow as solutions to their health. The reader should consult his or her medical health team or other competent professional before adopting any of the suggestions in this book, or drawing inferences from it. The authors and publisher are disclosing what has worked for them individually and specifically remove all responsibility for any liability, loss or risk personal or otherwise, which is incurred as a consequence, directly or indirectly, of the use and application of any of the contents of this book including and not limited to the reader stopping his or her personalized treatment without consulting with their professional medical team.

FOREWORD

Jack Canfield

I began my career as a History teacher in the inner city schools of Chicago where most of my students where under privileged and many struggled through school as a result of their circumstances at home. Several were the product of broken and dysfunctional homes and this provided me with a glimpse of how the emotional and mental wellbeing of many of these children would be forever affected by these circumstances. This was a story I knew well since I was also the product of a dysfunctional family with both of my parents being alcoholics and my father being physically abusive.

Later in my career, as a psychologist and psychotherapist, I got to see firsthand what emotionally and mentally unbalanced individuals go through on a daily basis and the effects mental illness can have when untreated. In many cases, mental illness had a devastating impact on their lives, their families, their community and ultimately, our society.

Yet, throughout the subsequent years of my career as an author, speaker, self-development trainer and self-esteem advocate, I had the privilege to come across thousands of people who, despite their circumstances, have been able to turn their lives around and begin a quest to not only improve their own lives but to also improve the lives of many around them through their personal experiences of survival and triumph.

These are the stories you will find in the book you are holding. *Faces of Mental Illness* is the work of 20 brave individuals who were invited and led by three of my students[1] to share their own personal experience with mental illness. Their intention is to break the silence about the illness; create awareness for families, loved ones and society; provide an honest and raw perspective of what living with a mental illness is like; end the stigma surrounding mental illness; and most importantly, bring hope to the millions of people around the world who are afflicted with a mental illness and who fight every single day to live a better life and be a positive influence and force in society.

Like me, each one of these individuals has found a way to thrive despite their circumstances. They have all experienced immense pain, struggled and fought with all they have against an illness that cannot be seen, continues to be misunderstood, and carries with it a high level of stigma. It is extraordinarily uplifting to follow their journey from feeling completely hopeless to reaching a place in their lives where happiness, joy and fulfillment have become possible.

Sadly, these are the stories we do not often hear, and they are the ones that must be heard so that we as a society have a better understanding of the signs, triggers, family life history and situations that can lead to mental illness, and to be informed and have access to all the treatments and resources that can lead us and our families to a life of mental health free from stigma and full of hope for the future.

As someone who has dedicated my entire life to self-improvement and as an author of the *Chicken Soup for the Soul*® series and

---

1—Claudia Fernandez-Niedzielski and Samantha Ruth are both Certified Trainers of The Success Principles™ and the Canfield Methodology, and Kate Butler is a student of my Breakthrough to Success Training. They are all #1 bestselling authors and transformational speakers reaching thousands with a message of hope for the future.

The Success Principles™, I am filled with joy reading the stories of these individuals who have overcome extreme odds, have learned how to cope with their illnesses, and have gone to live successful and fulfilling lives. And it is my hope that by reading these stories, you are able to find the way so that you too can do the same.

Jack Canfield, Coauthor of the *Chicken Soup for the Soul*®series and The Success Principles™: *How to Get from Where You Are to Where You Want to Be*

INTRODUCTION:

FACES OF MENTAL ILLNESS
OUR JOURNEY FROM STIGMA TO HEALTH

This book is about the many ways, shapes, forms, colors, faces, and stages, of how mental illness manifests in each one of us who have been dealt this card in the game of life.

It is the voice of many, who at one point have felt alone, discriminated, misunderstood, judged, stigmatized, unseen, unheard, wounded, and simply different from the rest of the world and yet have chosen to show up with all our imperfections and emotional struggles to make an impact on their lives, their communities, their families and ultimately create a totally different outcome from the one society has been taught to expect of anyone with a mental illness.

This is a project that carries not only hope for all those who are mentally ill but also delivers love, compassion and understanding to all the families, friends, significant others and communities who surround each one of us; for we also understand how difficult it can be to live with us and among us.

It is a way to shine a different light into a secret many of us carry and are extremely scared and ashamed to share with the rest of the world. It carries with it a huge responsibility, not only to ourselves and those we love; but to the world and the rest of humanity.

We trust you will join us on our quest to end the Stigma on Mental Illness.

Claudia Fernandez-Niedzielski
Samantha Ruth
Kate Butler

table of contents

Shapeshifter

Samantha Dee Niedzielski
(Daughter of Claudia Fernandez-Niedzielski)

I beat my chest for control
two fists kneading
the shapes of everything I've ever felt
for months, or days, or just minutes.
My moods shift like loose air
so I've stacked boulders
tied a something knot
around what's unruly.
And still ugly spills
from the thread and rock
into my lap
at the foot of my small mountain.
Day and night tumble
in the sky this repeats
I am upset, I am sad, I am happy, and
I am.
I will probably never stop stacking
or kneading will never stop feeling,
will need to remember
that I can leave my small mountain.
Let it become even smaller in the distance
let it be for a while
and when I return (because I always return)
I'll give it a name
and notice that my own two hands
are moving the boulders
& loosening the threads.

MY BIG SECRET

Claudia Fernandez-Niedzielski

It was November of 1994 when John and I met in Mexico City, where I am originally from. It was love at first sight, as he would later tell me and somehow I knew he meant it. We began dating just one week after we met and after one month of knowing each other, he invited me to visit him in Sacramento so that I could meet his family. This was moving very fast to say the least and it seemed serious enough that he wanted his family to meet me. I was extremely excited and said yes to his invitation. My father was not as pleased. The not so distant memories of what had happened to me the last time I had fallen in love with someone who lived so many miles away began to fill his mind with a terrifying fear.

Like any young girl in love would do when addressing her parent's concerns; I pushed them aside and told him that I was taking the past into account and left anyway. Somehow, I knew and felt that this time would be different.

I arrived in Sacramento just before New Year's Eve and after having a lovely day meeting his family and friends, I could not relax. My anxiety and nerves began to consume me. I had agreed to the visit and had done it knowing that this will be the best opportunity to share my huge and scary secret. It was a secret that could destroy it all and one I would later find out, exists in every family (including his own), but everyone is way too scared to talk about it.

There was no turning back and as we settled into a nice evening, I gathered all my courage and began by saying "John, there is something important you need to know, and after I tell you what I have to say, I will not blame you if you decide that this is just too much to take on. I will certainly understand." He really did not know what to say and I began to share my secret, my story.

I was an exchange student in Lester, Iowa during my senior year of High School in 1986. I was 18 years old, happy to be experiencing new things and happy to be away from home. It was not long after I arrived that I met someone special and fell deeply in love with him. We dated long distance for the following four years during which he traveled to Mexico to meet my family and I visited him in Iowa every summer. By the summer of 1991 he had become my obsession and the pain and sadness of being so far away (or so I thought) had become a deep agony and eventually an excruciating force that began to kill my spirit. I would lock myself in my room for hours on end. I stopped doing the things that were once fun for me. I would refuse to go out with my friends. I would find myself bursting into tears at work, while walking on the streets or while driving to and from work. I began to engage in reckless sexual behavior with men I would have never even considered dating at all before. I declined job offers that would have meant huge advancements in my career. I spent more money than I made until I came to the conclusion (on my very confused state) that this horrible experience was rooted in the fact that I was so far away from the man I desperately (and obsessively) loved and right there and then, I made the decision that the only way to end it all was to move to Iowa for good. I had no idea how wrong I was and no one in my family could have anticipated how cruel and devastating the truth of what was happening would come to be.

I arrived in Iowa in January of 1992 determined to begin my new life with the man I loved. Unfortunately, the time we had spent apart had not served us well and two weeks after I arrived in Iowa the relationship ended. It was not what I thought it would be and now I was left with a huge hole in my heart and still in a very fragile emotional state.

And then all hell broke loose. It was a cold, February night in Lester, Iowa in 1992 when the world as I knew it changed forever. I was staying with members of my American host parents and suddenly I was awakened by bright lights that begged me to follow them. I ran outside the house towards the church, then ran back to the home of my American host parents' family as I desperately tried to escape the voices and steps of those I could swear were chasing me. As I entered the empty house (my host family was on vacation), I made a mess. I removed all the unloaded guns from the gun case, removed all my clothes from the drawers, decided to take a bath and threw pillows, comforters, and sheets out of the window and jumped out of the one-and-a-half story house, fully naked, to escape from the voices. I don't know how long I ran around the small town. They would later tell me that I ended up knocking on someone's door in the very early hours of the morning and that soon after I was hospitalized at a Psychiatry Hospital in South Dakota. The doctors called "it" a full-blown psychotic episode; one that would require the use of a straight-jacket, heavy medications, and a padded cell to avoid self-harm and harm to others. The diagnosis (one that would later be changed) was schizophrenia. I cannot begin to imagine what my parents felt when they got that call. What followed was a terrifying and very dark time in my family's life. It was true that I was depressed before I left Mexico and my parents could see I was not happy, but this was too much and too hard to understand.

My dad immediately flew to South Dakota to bring me back home, although it would be a long time before I was truly home.

I arrived at the Mexican Institute of Psychiatry in Mexico City, where my entire family was interviewed, and after several tests my family would hear the correct diagnosis for the first time. "Claudia has Bipolar disorder," my doctor said. And it seems that the psychotic episode she has suffered has severely damaged her emotional compass and the person she truly is. It would take six more months of hospitalization with 24/7 care by family members, while my doctor experimented with all sorts of medication and therapy. My case was so severe that it was brought up to the attention of the board of psychiatry and it would become a case study with no favorable results. My parents were driven to such despair that at one point, they pleaded for God to take me if this was the way I was going to be for the rest of my life.

Life, God, the Universe, destiny or whatever you would want to call it, I believe had a different plan for my life and it came in the way of one of the most misunderstood treatments for mental illness.

As a last resource, my doctor suggested she would try electro convulsive (or electro shock) therapy, which is considered a highly controversial treatment. This meant my brain would be rebutted like you rebut a computer through shocks of electricity. There were huge risks, but there was nothing more to lose at that point and at least my parents would know they had done everything they could within their reach. If successful, I would at least be present somewhat, somehow. If not, my life and that of my entire family would never be the same. Right after the 1st session we all knew this was the beginning of my recovery. I could remember places I had been and when I communicated my sentences made sense. I looked at my parents in their eyes and this time they could see that my spirit was back, this was truly a total success. I can only imagine how much relief and joy my parents felt on that day. It took a total of 10 sessions to get me out of the darkness I had been in. I was back as the person you see right now, although my life had been changed forever and there would be hurdles and obstacles in the future, since I would always live with Bipolar Disorder."

There it was. I had shared my deepest big secret and was now sobbing. John sat there quietly and I truly would not have blamed him if he would have said this was more than he could handle in a relationship and yet, as I finished sharing my story, he wiped my tears and said, "Thank you so much for sharing this with me and know that I love you and have loved you since the day I met you and I do not care about this at all. We will work through it and will handle it together."

It would truly be a fairy tale if I told you that everything has been rainbows and butterflies since that day and through our 27 years of marriage, but it would also be a huge lie. His ignorance at the time for what this diagnosis truly meant was bigger than he had thought. How could he know any different since when he met me there was no visible indication that I was ill and through medication and regular visits to my doctor, I was doing extremely well? How could he have known that through the years we have been married, there would be many times where I would be totally absent (emotionally) and others where I would be extremely happy and high as a kite on life with no way to get me down? His deep love and understanding has kept him with me through these highs and lows as I continue to live with Bipolar disorder or Manic-Depressive Illness.

He would soon discover that during the very highs, which are the manic episodes, I can stay awake for hours and work on 10 projects at a time without feeling tired, without needing sleep or food, and the ideas and creativity during these periods come with such a furious force that I feel like I could almost take the world in my hands and rebuild it in just one day and there is nothing, absolutely nothing I cannot do and the sun shines ever so brightly creating an euphoria I can hardly contained inside. Then the light disappears completely during the lows, which are the depressive episodes. As the darkness sets it and covers everything around me my energy is gone, my positive outlook on life is no longer there, the immense sadness I experience crushes my heart and my vitality and desire to continue on is completely non-existent. The pain you feel inside is the size of the ocean and there is nothing that can get it to disappear.

I no longer experience these drastic changes as I fully understand that my body needs medication and occasional therapy to thrive. Despite it all, I stand before you proud to be who I am, for I have so much I have accomplished and plenty more to do. I have been married for almost 27 years. I have two children whom I love with all my heart. I have practiced Real Estate successfully for the last 15 years. I have managed a few Real Estate offices and I have trained other individuals in my field. I have become a #1 International Best Selling author*. I am a Jack Canfield Success Principles Certified Trainer and most of the time I perform at a very high level.

Meeting Jack Canfield in 2015 would ignite a huge desire to share my story with others to positively impact their lives and provide hope and understanding for and of mental illness. Through applying many of his Principles, I followed my desire and became a Mental Health advocate and speaker and it is because of that first step that the book you are holding in your hands became a reality. It is such a wonder that what I feared the most at one point, which was sharing my story, would become such a positive force of change and hope for so many.

It has not been easy, but having full understanding of my illness, full recognition of my triggers, and by staying under the supervision of my doctor, it has been absolutely POSSIBLE to not just live . . . but thrive with a mental illness. I am living proof that there is much more to us than our madness and that life is so much brighter because we are in it!

Women Who Illuminate and *Women Who Rise*

ABOUT CLAUDIA FERNANDEZ-NIEDZIELSKI

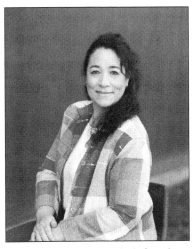

Claudia became obsessed with positive information and positive quotes after her father introduced her and her brothers to books that would inspire them to always strive to be the best they could be.

Claudia is a fighter, a survivor and a woman who has learned to thrive despite the many challenges she has faced. She loves her parents, brothers, children, husband and extended family with all her heart and continues to learn how to live a life full of passion and in full harmony with herself. She has a genuine and profound impact on others as she mentors and leads them to live life to the fullest and shares the tools she has utilized on her own personal search for meaning, self-discovery, understanding and compassion for herself and others and her deep self-worth.

One of her desires was to impact the lives of others living with a Mental Illness through education and sharing her own story of survival and resilience. In 2015, this desire would lead her to join "Stigma Sacramento Speakers Bureau", a non-profit organization in Sacramento fully dedicated to the education of the community as to what mental illness truly is with the goal to stop the stigma on mental illness, create awareness, provide resources and give hope! In the last 6 years, she has spoken to thousands of people in Sacramento, has appeared on Fox News and has been a radio show guest as an advocate for mental illness.

Claudia is an Amazon #1 International best-selling author*, a transformational speaker, a small business consultant and a Real Estate Professional. She is a Jack Canfield Success Principles® Certified Associate Trainer and a Barrett Value Center® Certified Practitioner and Consultant.

*Women Who Illuminate and Women Who Rise

To learn more about Claudia Fernandez-Niedzielski, you can visit her website at:www.ClaudiaImpactsLives.com

To book Claudia as a speaker or work with her, please contact her directly at:

ClaudiaImpactsLives@gmail.com
(916) 248-3004 Direct

BECOMING RUTHLESS

Samantha Ruth

Memorial Day, 1997. I don't remember where I was going, but I absolutely remember that it's the day I got in my first car accident. I was 23 and traumatized. So much so that I refused to drive afterwards. My mom, the sweetest woman on the planet, secretly rented a car for me and left me at Enterprise so I'd have to drive myself home. I was pisssssed off, to put it mildly.

I still "put my foot down" and refused to drive on the expressway, because that's where my accident happened. I took the main roads wherever I had to go, no matter how much longer it took me. Mind you, this all seemed completely logical and rational to me at the time. Laugh if you must, but I'm being one hundred percent serious.

As if this wasn't enough for my young, naive self to deal with, just less than two weeks later, on Father's Day, a power line fell across the fence and in my backyard. I'll explain.

I was lying out, reading and enjoying a typical Sunday with my dog, Harlie, who was an itty bitty thing at the time. Out of the blue, Harlie started barking incessantly and looking up at what I thought could only be our tree. I stood up and saw what I thought was a large tree branch falling. I grabbed Harlie and ran in my house only to hear the most insane noises, including my neighbors screaming. Still holding onto Harlie, I grabbed my keys (because that's what seemed necessary at the time) and I ran out the front door (in only my bathing suit still) where I was greeted by neighbors rushing to see if I was ok.

"Thank goodness you went inside and out the front door rather than going out through your fence. You would have been electrocuted." Lovely.

Smoke. Sirens. Someone giving me clothes to cover up. I wasn't even wearing shoes. Firemen running around frantically. They wouldn't let me back inside because the downed power line had caused an electrical fire in my house.

I don't remember the rest. My parents must have rushed over, although this was before cell phones so a neighbor must have called them. Still mentally recovering from the car accident, this pushed me over the edge.

I started rearranging furniture in the middle of the night, in case I needed a rapid escape plan. I hardly slept, and if I did, I'd wake in a panic. It sounds ridiculous, I know, but it's really how I was living. Lists and more lists. Escape plans. Panic. Lots and lots of panic.

This continued until I just broke down one day while at grad school. The thing about becoming a psychologist is that you're required to go through ALL the therapy yourself. Thank God! It took my classmates and my professor's prodding for me to finally open up and talk honestly about what I was dealing with.

Hello? I'm in school to become a psychologist and I didn't even recognize my own PTSD. The more I talked, the more I felt, and it seemed as if I was just one big walking emotion.

I'd never had therapy at this point, so this was my first time actually dealing with "my stuff" and hearing other perspectives and input. Usually it was just me and the mean girls in my head, pointing out all of my flaws, mistakes, and quirks.

Now I had people providing support, encouragement, and alternative opinions, the most popular of which was that I'd been living with anxiety for years. I was looking at myself in an entirely new way, because this was truly a newsflash to me.

Don't get me wrong, I always knew I was different. From my family. From my friends. From everyone. You would never have known by looking at me, but I ALWAYS felt like the odd one out. The black sheep. The one that didn't belong. I had never connected my inner turmoil to any of this until now. That's the thing with invisible illnesses. You can be at war on the inside and look completely fine to the rest of the world. And it's not like I was the girl shaking in the corner with anxiety.

I was pretty much the exact opposite. Sports. Plays. Clubs. You name it, I was involved. None of that ever interfered with my grades or my jobs. Can we say overachiever altogether now?

But this was the first time I was looking at WHY I was such an overachiever. Why did I need to do one more thing and then one more? It was my way of quieting the noise. Of quieting those mean girls in my head, or should I say my attempt to quiet them.

I've had anxiety my entire life, but I was just now seeing it. Seeing Little Girl Sam, organizing anything and everything, including disorganizing only to reorganize again.

All the years of being told to shake it off and pull myself together, because something must be wrong with me, right? All the years of being called too sensitive. All the years of thinking. And thinking. And rethinking. Overthinking.

Needless to say, this was a new beginning for me and especially for my relationship with myself. I started therapy. I started taking medication. I started learning how to manage my anxiety. I started learning the importance of being honest about my anxiety, with myself and with others.

That doesn't mean it was always well received or even understood. For that matter, it wasn't easy for me on a personal level either. I had to spend a lot of time working on accepting the fact that I have anxiety. Because this world we live in stigmatizes mental illness. And judges. And, and, and . . . Because I've been taught, on the court and in life, to push through. Because my dad is a doctor and psychology is anything but scientific.

And even though I understood intellectually that it's the world with the ass backwards assumption that mental illness equals bad, emotionally coming to terms with the fact that this now included me was an entirely different matter altogether. And an ongoing process.

Add to that the fact that anxiety is very regularly poo pooed. "Just don't worry about it." "It will be fine." "Calm down." And millions of other comments implying that it's a choice or that we can just turn it off like a switch.

For years this combination had me on a mission "to "fix it.". Even during the stretches when I had minimal anxiety, I would continue working on how to fix it for the next time. Because there's always a next time. Life is full of ups and downs and triggers.

But I'm that Type A girl, remember? Overachieving. Adding more to my resume. Pushing through. So whenever I did struggle, the rest of the world had no idea. I was a great student, and I had learned to put my anxiety in a private place—where it belonged.

There were situations and people I did choose to share my anxiety with. And many were supportive. Those who weren't helped me become even more passionate about my mission to change the way the world views mental illness.

But there were still just as many people and situations I didn't share my anxiety with. Maybe it was the pressure of being a psychologist and being expected to have it all together, all the time. Maybe it was my fear of people's reactions. Of changing people's opinions of me.

When asked by these people how I was doing, I always answered with "fine" or "great." I put on this pretense while the war was raging on the inside. It's invisible, remember? I wasn't aware of this then. I wasn't consciously creating these two separate worlds, but looking back I can see it so vividly.

I had my thriving psychology practice, a wonderful family, amazing friends, a house, a fur baby . . . A great life. And I held my anxiety in its own private place—where it belonged.

It would pop up at expected times, like in really big crowds. Or when my dad became sick. I must make a side note here and tell you that I was told to pull myself together. By my extended family and the people I trust the most, again making me question myself when in reality I was having the healthiest reaction of everyone involved!

That's the world we live in, but that doesn't make it right. If only I knew this then. Ok, back to my anxiety and the fact that it popped up due to my circumstances. Like moving across the country to marry my soulmate. And driving. Always driving!

Then there were the unexpected times my anxiety would make an appearance. The times without a clear triggering incident. Because that's what anxiety does. It has a mind of its own and it shows up whenever and wherever, with or without warning. And I'd find myself wondering why, when things were great and I had so much to be grateful for, my anxiety would show up. I now know that's just what it does, but in the thick of it, you just have more to think (and rethink) about.

So I navigated and used my tools. I helped so many others work through their anxiety. I found healthy outlets, like working out and changing my nutrition, all of which helped me manage my anxiety even better. I lived life successfully . . . with my anxiety in its own, private place—where it belonged.

I've had anxiety my entire life, but it took losing my husband for me to truly understand it and learn how to thrive with it . . . in a non-separate place, if you will. In a "public" place.

Less than four years ago, I lost my everything. I was deep in grief, and my anxiety reached levels I'd never before experienced. It was at an all-time high while I was living through the absolute worst time of my life.

I was in so much pain that I just didn't care. I didn't care about those two worlds, the one for me and the other for my anxiety. I didn't care what people's reactions may or may not be. I didn't care if it made them uncomfortable. I didn't care if they saw me in a new light. I just didn't care.

Instead of fighting it or hiding it, I began fully embracing it. Owning it. Sharing about it with others. And the most amazing thing happened. I could breathe. Like that first breath of fresh morning air, I could really and fully breathe.

All these years I'd been doing what the world expected of me. But now I could see that THAT was the problem.

Everything began to shift from this point forward. Yes, I was living through my absolute nightmare of losing Jim. But in my grief, I was finding myself. Finding my voice. Finding my purpose in this life without Jim by my side. Becoming Ruthless!

Jim was the one person who truly loved and accepted me for me. All of me. Exactly as I am. And without him, I was fully learning to accept me for me. Exactly as I am. I thought I had worked on this in the past, but now I could see that I had only accepted parts of myself.

I'm not saying my anxiety is gone. It's still a part of me. It's a part I've learned to see as a gift. It makes me more sensitive to others and to their emotions. It looks out for me.

It's a part of me that I not only accept . . . it's also a part of me I embrace. I'm open and honest with myself and with the world. For several reasons.

It's part of living successfully with anxiety. Hiding. Fighting. Resisting. That only makes it worse. It might make some people uncomfortable, but let me be very clear, that's their issue, not mine. That's a reflection of themselves, not of myself.

It's also my way of letting others know that You Are Not Alone. You don't need to struggle alone. Mental illness can be isolating and that's wrong! I want you to know that you need others. You need others who get it. Period.

It's part of Becoming Ruthless . . . which is another story

entirely! Suffice it to say that it's about being unapologetically me. It's about being true to myself and my intuition. It's about using my voice. It's about turning my perceived weaknesses into my biggest strengths. Such as my anxiety. So this negativity-charged word now has the most positive meaning. Just like Mental Illness—once you embrace it. Ruthlessly.

It's also my way of making noise and working to break stigmas and change the way the world views mental illness. Silence is the enemy. We need to normalize these conversations so that people can get the help they need AND deserve.

I've had anxiety my entire life, and it makes me, ME.

ABOUT SAMANTHA RUTH

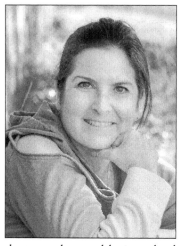

Samantha is a Psychologist, Speaker, Best Selling Author, and the Proud Founder of Griefhab, a 24/7 support community open to anyone who has experienced a loss. She helps people around the world turn their pain into their power by guiding them to be their true selves, not who they think they need to be, by embracing their differences and by living life on their own terms.

Samantha's mission is to change the way the world views both grief and mental health, so people can speak about whatever issues they have and get the help they not only need, but deserve, without fear of judgment, labels, and repercussions.

In her free time, you can find Samantha with her pups on one of their outdoor adventures. Music fuels Samantha's soul, family means everything to her, and honoring her late husband, Jim, and making him proud gives her life daily purpose.

You can work with Samantha individually, in one of her exclusive groups, or you can have her speak at your event or organization. Contact Samantha to determine what's best for you at sam@samantharuth.com.

www.samantharuth.com

https://www.facebook.com/samanthamruth

https://www.linkedin.com/in/samanthamruth

https://www.instagram.com/samanthamruth

https:/www.Twitter.com/Samanthamruth

https://www.facebook.com/groups/griefhab7

https://podcasts.apple.com/us/podcast/the-be-ruthless-show/id1554585454

https://www.joinclubhouse.com/@samantharuth

"17"

Kate Butler

When I was 17-years-old my dear friend, Meghan, took her own life.

It was the summer after our senior year of high school. The sun was hot, the air was salty and our dreams for the future were bright, or so it seemed. Having grown up in Southern New Jersey, we spent our summers at the Jersey Shore. There were a couple rented beach houses where our group of friends hung out most weekends, and Meghan was a staple in one of those houses. I remember those summer nights so clearly.

We would sit around as a group, in some sort of makeshift circle and slightly reminiscence, but mostly forward hope. Looking back I can see how uncomfortable Meghan would get when the conversations would change to college and the different paths we would all be taking soon. She would shift in her seat and not really engage. It wasn't anything drastic, but even at that age I could intuitively pick up on the emotions of others, and I knew something was not quite right. Yet, I had no frame of reference for just how bad it was for her.

I was at my parents' shore house when I received "the call" and I was stunned to my core. Meghan had hung herself in her parent's garage. I never knew darkness of this depth until this moment. It was like someone had pulled back the curtain of a deep, dark, endless hole of pain. This wasn't just any hole; this hole had sharp, slimy, jagged, unforgiving teeth that made up the edges of this tunnel. The tunnel had a force that pulled you into its spiral that was nearly impossible to fight. This was my very first experience with the tunnel of despair. Up until this point I would play with the edges of these feelings, but I never even conceived there was a real option of crossing to the other side. Once Meghan took that leap, I realized this was a very real, painful reality, that these weren't edges to keep us in, but these were actually cliffs of darkness that with one slip, could have us fall into the darkness forever.

There were very few people I spoke to about this new awareness I was experiencing. Quite frankly, I am not sure I had the language at 17 to even articulate all that I was thinking or feeling. But it was the first time in my life I had felt that level of hopelessness.

A few months later, our group of friends, including myself, was off to college to start our new journeys. Although I was hours and miles and states away from this tragedy, it always stayed very close to my heart as a reminder of just how close the edge of that cliff could be.

Time went on. I did not forget, but I did begin to heal.

As I entered into adulthood, I encountered more death and life altering events, but nothing that hit me quite as tragic as what my dear friend experienced. As I lived through these other experiences, I deduced that I had developed enough coping skills to process the tough experiences without ever taking me back to that dark spiraling tunnel again.

After college I moved to California from the East Coast, a lifelong dream come true. I found a job that I loved and was a complete rock star at that company, becoming the youngest person at that time in an executive position where I was running a multi-million dollar office at 24-years-old. I was on the brink of massive success and loving life. It was at this time that I also met my husband, Mel. He was from the East Coast, as well, and we hit it off instantly. He was only supposed to be in California for six weeks for a project he was working on. Those six weeks became six months, and then almost a year. Eventually he had to return back to his work on the East Coast. At this point, I had lived in California for seven years and I was ready for something new. Mel and I knew we wanted to take our relationship to the next level and we both decided we wanted to do that on the East Coast near both of our families. We got married a year later, and were expecting our first child a year after that. This was the highest point in my life thus far. I was flying high.

We moved into our dream house when I was 7-months pregnant with Bella, our first daughter. Nesting was in full effect to get everything set and ready for the arrival of our precious baby.

We didn't find out the gender and I desperately wanted a girl. So I convinced myself I was having a boy and that I was happy about it so I wouldn't be disappointed. Oh, the games we play with ourselves when we are still evolving in our personal growth!

Bella arrived on her due date (as did my second daughter Livie, two and half years later) and she was the biggest shock of my life. When the doctor said it was a girl and I heard that first cry, I released every emotion I had built up during the pregnancy and it all came out in that moment. I was sobbing hysterically. The doctor looked at my husband in shock and said "Is she ok?" Mel said, "Yes, she's just really, really happy." And I was. I couldn't talk and I could barely breathe, but this was the happiest moment of my life.

I was beyond exhausted in the hospital, getting sleep in increments of 1-2 hours at a time. I was still in the bliss of the baby bubble, but I was growing weak and weary with the lack of sleep and the toll of what my body had just gone through. It was all catching up with me.

It was release day from the hospital and it was time to get ready to go home. I brought my bag of clothes into the bathroom to change out of the nursing gown I had been wearing. I attempted to put on my pants and they didn't make it up past my thighs. I was so confused. I tried on my shirt and I couldn't get it over my chest. What the heck? It had never occurred to me that my regular clothes wouldn't just fit again after having a baby. Why didn't anyone tell me this? Was it because I was the only one who still needed to wear maternity clothes leaving the hospital? I was so embarrassed and felt humiliated as I asked my husband to hand me the maternity clothes I had come to the hospital in. He asked unknowingly, "Don't you have your clothes bag in there?" I snapped. I went into a rage. I barked something back. I went into hysterics. And I saw the black tunnel . . . again . . . for the first time in years. This was way more than hormones being out of whack. I went to a dark place and fast. I was so scared of that vision of the tunnel that I snapped myself out of it.

What had just happened?

I got myself together, got dressed in my maternity clothes and forced myself to get back into that baby bubble. It was going to take some intense effort, but I was determined to get back to that blissful place.

By the time we got home I had settled down. I was getting back into the bubble.

A few weeks later I took Bella to a doctor's appointment and he told me that Bella had lost weight. And in no uncertain terms also told me that if I was determined to continue nursing that I was basically choosing to starve my baby.

I got in the car and lost it.

I was a monster who was hurting my baby. I hated myself.

The tunnel was back.

A few weeks later, having not given up because I was convinced I was doing the right thing for my baby, Bella was having trouble latching and I hadn't slept for more than a few hours in a row now for over a month. I was trying to feed her and she was hysterically crying. I started hysterically crying. The more upset I got, the more upset she got.

I was a complete failure and sorry excuse for a mom.

The tunnel was back.

When Bella was about 4 months old, we started to feel the pressure of money being really tight. We had agreed I would resign from my corporate position to stay home with Bella. We had also agreed that our spending would have to remain very controlled in order for that to work. I had bought Bella some baby outfits for a photo session and charged it. Mel came home from work and asked me about the charges and how we were going to pay for it.

I exploded.

I was now a failure as a wife. Not only am I a complete failure as a mom, but now I don't contribute anything financially to the family either. I am worthless.

The tunnel was back.

This pattern went on, viciously, only getting worse throughout the first year of Bella's life.

The tunnel was never far away. When I was alone, when I allowed myself to be honest with my thoughts . . . I was IN the tunnel. I had entered it and I would step down and down and see how far into despair I could go. It was like a punishment to myself for not being good enough. I didn't deserve to be happy. I didn't deserve the good. I deserved the tunnel.

My feelings of unworthiness started to show up in every area of my life. I began to self-sabotage career opportunities, friendships, family relationships and even my marriage. Thankfully my husband somehow was able to bear with me and did not allow this to happen.

I now know this was severe postpartum depression, but I didn't even have that language when I was going through it. Sure I had heard of it before, but I never explored it or really understood it.

I had never had conversations about it and certainly no one ever said, this is how you may feel or this is what you may look out for.

My depression never had anything to do with my baby. I always loved, adored and cherished every single moment with her. In fact, she was my life line.

My depression was all internalized and it was all about me. It was self-loathing at its finest. I hated myself, not anyone else.

There were many times it came out in ways that appeared to be about other people, but these were all forms of self-sabotage. These were all ways of making sure I destroyed anything good in my life, because deep down I didn't believe I deserved to have it. Except for my baby, she was perfect, she was my miracle. She was the one thing that got all my pure love and grace. She was off limits. I'm not sure how in the world I made that distinction, but I am oh so grateful that I did. It was never about anyone else, it was always about my own inner demons.

The turning point was right before my 31st birthday. Bella was about 9 months old at the time. I started to get this idea that I wanted to look and feel my best on my birthday. At first I told myself it wasn't possible and stuffed the thoughts down. But one day when it came up, I clung to it. It was my first miracle, besides Bella, in a long time. I held onto that opening for dear life. It was like I was holding onto this rope of light that was going to pull me out of the tunnel. But there was a catch, I had to be strong enough to climb up this rope and pull myself up or I would fall back into the spiral forever.

As I started to climb that rope of light, I began to do things for myself. They started very small. I started to care about what I ate. I took the time to notice how the food made me feel. I then started to take yoga classes. These made me feel even better. Yoga opened me up to meditation and this is really what shifted everything for me.

I started to explore meditation and everything I read said that consistent meditation could be transformational. Most recommended a consistent practice for 30 days to see those types of results.

Well I was in the market for a transformation so I decided to put that challenge to the test.

Even the fact that I was able to take on this challenge was another miracle moment in my life. I had begun stacking my chips in a new direction. For almost a year, I had stacked all of my chips on the path of self-sabotage, self-loathing and unworthiness. When I began stacking in feelings of well-being, slivers of joy and feeling energized, it allowed me to keep saying yes to things on this new path.

About three weeks into my consistent meditation practice something did happen. I started to feel this warmth bubble up from the center of my body. It began to travel up my spine all the way to the top of my head and also down my legs all the way to the toes of my feet. I sat with this feeling for many, many minutes. About a half hour later when I opened my eyes I realized this was the first time in my life I had ever experienced the feeling of true inner peace.

Up until this point in my life, even when I was happy or at my highest of highs, those feelings were always associated with something outside of myself. A job, or promotion, or success of some sort, a relationship or an event. For the first time in my life I had accessed and fully experienced inner joy and inner peace from a place deep inside of me. I felt elation. This was an unparalleled feeling. But more than that, it was an opening of consciousness that would ultimately help me arrive at a new way of thinking.

I began to think, if this were possible, what else could be possible? And this was the opening I needed to truly begin my healing journey. Another miracle moment in my life.

I began to develop my own practices of meditation, journaling with God, divine co-creation methods and a few other tools that have not only helped me heal, but have completely transformed my life.

The tunnel is now distant. I know it still exists, but my daily practices keep me operating in a place where, when the tunnel gets close, I understand the tools that will help pull me out with the rope of light.

It's not a perfect science, but it is what works for me.

That moment when I was 17 was an opening into a world I didn't know existed. And once you know, you can't unknow. That moment when I was 31 was an opening into a world that I didn't know existed. And once you know, you can't unknow.

Life is full of opening moments and in each one we are given the power to choose. On some days that choice may be a baby step and on other days it may be a giant leap. I always remind myself where I am stacking my chips. My desire is to have more chips stacked on this path of joy and fulfillment, which ultimately allows me to live out my life purpose. When we are able to live from this place, show up for other people and pour into other people, life becomes so much richer. So some days I don't stack the chips for me, I stack the chips for them.

I started to recognize that the strength of the light was just as powerful as the strength of despair. I get to choose. They both still exist, but I have the power to choose. This awareness is nothing short of the greatest miracle in my life, because I truly believe it is what saved me and what continues to save me every day.

ABOUT KATE BUTLER

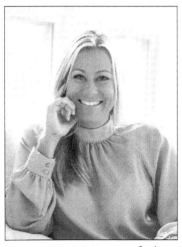

Kate Butler is a TV Host, Publisher, #1 International Best-selling Author and Speaker. Kate is the host of the TV Show, "Where It's All Possible" which streams on Roku. She is also creator of the *Inspired Impact Book Series*, a #1 International Best-selling Series that has published over 300 authors. Kate focuses on taking your story and bringing it to life in a best-selling book . . . this is her specialty!

As a CPSC, Certified Professional Success Coach, she offers dynamic live and digital programs creating transformational experiences to ultimately help clients reach their greatest potential and live out their dreams, including becoming a #1 Best-selling Author through her mentorship. Kate believes in learning the tools to help create those "Made For Moments" in your life. Her passion is teaching others how to activate their authentic mission, share it for massive impact while also creating a lucrative business.

Kate's expertise has been featured on Fox 29, GoodDay Philadelphia, HBO, PHL 17, Roku the RVN network and many more tv and radio platforms.

Kate offers a variety of free tools on her website to help you get clear on what you want and also to show you the path to make it possible. Visit www.katebutlerbooks.com

Connect with Kate to learn more about how you can achieve your ultimate potential at www.katebutlerbooks.com.

THE SOUR PATCH KID

Sarah Abbott

My whole life I have been known to be somewhat of a Sour Patch Kid. You know; first they are sour . . . then they are sweet! The commercials for these delicious bipolar treats often explained me perfectly. You would see these little gummies doing something extremely sour (like cut off a little girl's ponytail), then recover with something really sweet (like drop the scissors and reach out for a hug). But, when living between states of severe depression and severe mania, how could I not relate to these commercials? Especially when trying to live with an ignored diagnosis, a family skeptical of mental illness's legitimacy, and no medication to help. I have been struggling with bipolar disorder since an early age; however, I have not been actually living/thriving with it until more recently. I was first diagnosed at around age 15, but did not get any help or treatment until I was in my thirties.

I remember feeling things in extremes since I was about 10 or so and I was often labeled as being 'too sensitive,' 'dramatic,' or 'impulsive.' I lived in two worlds. First, a state of mania where everything was nonstop, my energy was off the charts, and everything felt relatively 'awesome'. I was more talkative, energetic, promiscuous, and would do almost everything in excess. This included drugs/alcohol, going out, gambling, cleaning, and running a mile a minute. Others would often assume that I was on cocaine or some other 'upper' substance, so I was accused of having a drug problem quite often. In reality, I was simply bouncing between mania and depression. Which brings me to the other state I would often live in—depression. During these times it was hard to do anything, including getting up and interacting at any capacity. I would become extremely distant, have no energy, be very irritable, and literally nothing was okay, everything sucked! I do not remember ever feeling content, balanced, or any sense of normalcy.

Growing up I was the loud child, the super dramatic and sensitive black sheep. I was unpredictable and impulsive. I had a hard time paying attention, but was still highly successful at almost anything I actually committed to. I was either excelling and achieving awards or getting a phone call home every day for one thing or another. I often had a hard time maintaining relationships and never really felt I was 'a part' of anything. I often felt alone and misunderstood. I remember realizing at an early age that I felt things differently than others. I did not have 'normal' feelings and moods. Things would make me SUPER sad, or SUPER happy, or SUPER angry, and I would become whatever I was feeling. More often than not I was getting into some sort of trouble and had someone upset with me for something.

As things progressed into my teenage years, I began to try and control my emotions by self-medicating. If I were feeling over irritable and energized, full of anxiety, I would take some sort of downer to calm myself down. If I were feeling down, sad, hopeless, and restless, I would take some sort of upper to try and get some energy to 'snap out of it'. This did not always mean illegal drugs though, sometimes it was as simple as a bunch of energy drinks or smoking cigarettes. I was constantly trying to feel some sort of contentment, and it felt like the more I tried to find and explain myself, the more misunderstood I became. This led to the determination that Sarah must be a drug addict. This led to me being sent to several inpatient drug programs and doing a couple of stints in mental institutions. I even spent four years in a program that was later deemed by the state as a cult! I was diagnosed with many different things during this time (including bipolar) and tried many medications. Nothing stuck.

As things progressed into my early adulthood, I had a hard time keeping a job or having relationships, and I had several breakdowns. I would become so overwhelmed by my emotions and had nobody who understood me. At the time everyone was thinking I was just a lost cause and a druggie. My breakdowns would usually end with me hurting myself in some regard, most dangerously by physically cutting myself. Somehow it made sense to me if I could 'see' the pain I had inside represented by this cut, and I could watch that heal, I was also healing my unseen pain inside. This obviously never worked and often made me only appear to be unstable and 'crazy'. Which is a term that I have always struggled with because I regularly felt that I was losing my mind!

As I got older, life went on as 'normal' as possible, and I really tried to do 'normal' things. Most of the time this was just to please other people and appear that everything was okay (in my family that was silently expected). I got married, had a couple of kiddos, got my GED, and was working a decent job. I still struggled with mania and depression though and it became harder and harder to maintain my life. Things progressed and I eventually lost my job, went through a very messy and abusive divorce, and started living more recklessly again. Any time I did not have my kids, I was going out being careless or living in my dark bedroom. When I had my kids, I would occupy our time full of crafts and fun things to try and avoid getting stuck in my feelings.

As you can imagine, things could only progressively get worse the longer I tried to self-manage a medical condition, a mental illness. I began to be even more inconsistent and started to see the effect I was having on others in my life, especially my children.

I can imagine that everyone felt they had to walk on eggshells with me as I was so unpredictable—you never knew what you would get with me. I decided in my early thirties that something had to change and I knew that there was no way that life was supposed to be so difficult on a daily basis. I went and saw a psychologist (which was obviously nothing knew), but this time it was different. I was open and ready to understand what was going on with me and willing to do whatever it took to get better. It was at this time that I was re-diagnosed. I was diagnosed with Bipolar Disorder II, A.D.D, and anxiety, with some PTSD from my past traumas. I began the trial-and-error process for finding what medications and therapies worked for me. We went through a good 6-8 months of trying different medications and doing therapy once a week.

I remember having so many mixed feelings! Part of me felt so relieved and excited that I found out what my diagnosis was, and I could now get help—life was actually super simple and beautiful. The other part of me felt so sad that my life could have been better so much sooner, and I was super depressed that I suffered so long when treatment was right there the whole time. We found a combination of medication and treatment that worked for me. I was taking two mood stabilizers for Bipolar, one medication for A.D.D, and had some anxiety meds I would take as needed. I was speaking to my medication manager once a month and everything in life was SO much better! I was content, life made sense, my moods were managed, and I was thriving! I had the same job, great relationships, and while I still experienced highs and lows, they were manageable and did not take over my being.

So, here we were, age 36, thriving and living life. Then what happens? Well, I started feeling overwhelmed with having to take medication every day and I felt crazy again. I was exhausted from all the work I'd put in for over three years and made the GREAT decision that I was better and didn't need all these meds. I stopped taking them all, cold turkey. This ended up being a terrible decision! After about a month, I had a severe mental breakdown that ended up with me pulling a knife on myself, my boyfriend getting injured by the same knife, being arrested, and going through a year of domestic violence classes. Not to mention the huge financial impact this had and the effect that this had on my job as well. Things fell apart so quickly, and I was right back at what felt like the beginning.

I had now seen what life could be, and I had actually lived it. I was thriving for years. So despite this set back, I decided I wanted my life back and knew what I needed to do to get there. I picked myself up, got back on my meds, and practiced intense self-love. I did the work needed, took accountability, and realized that I was not crazy. I live with a mental illness. As far as the meds? I realized that if I had a heart condition, I would take meds to prevent a heart attack, so why was taking meds for this condition any different? I realized that this illness was not a curse that would take my life, but rather a condition that if treated, would empower me to be an even better person!

It has been over a year now since that incident and things are so good. I still have my bad days, but they do not define my life. Life is beautiful and I am not defined by my illness. I am not damaged goods. For so long I felt insecure or embarrassed that I was bipolar. I would get nervous for people to find out and would try to keep it a secret. When I would find the courage to let someone know, I would either get a sad response like "Oh no, you have bipolar? I am so sorry, that is so sad. I feel so bad for you," or I'd get a surprised and concerned reaction like "What? You have bipolar? Are you going to flip out on me? Let's keep this between us." It was like a big secret that I should be ashamed of and I definitely should not be trusted because I could lose it at any moment! Watch out world!

Well neither reaction is appropriate, it is caused by a stigmatism—a false perception of mental illness. I am no longer ashamed. I am proud to have bipolar. I operate the same, if not better, than most of the population! I am a good person, great Mom, excellent employee, loyal friend, and have mentored several other people struggling with mental illness and/or addiction. I have taught at prisons, volunteered as a life coach, and I am a reiki practitioner as well. I have an immense love for life and people! I have learned that I still have a love/hate relationship with bipolar and on my low days it is important to be vulnerable, honest, and communicate with my support system and on my manic days I utilize the energy constructively by creating (I am an artist as well), doing active things, and avoiding things that I could become obsessive about. I have learned not only how to live with my illness, but to actually thrive and live a life I love!

ABOUT SARAH ABBOTT

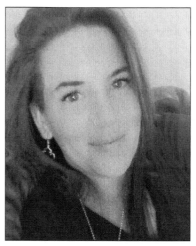

Sarah is an artist and mother of two with a career in the electronics industry. She has a genuine love for people and all things creative. Diagnosed with Bipolar Disorder, A.D.D., and Anxiety she thrives in Denver, Colorado working full time as an Account Manager. Sarah loves spending time with her two boys, Ethan 12 and Logan 10, as they are her world. She enjoys being outdoors, anything artistic, and truly gets absorbed in helping others. She is a certified Reiki practitioner and is working towards a psychology degree, with the hopes of one day helping others full time. She makes it a point to surround herself with fun and laughter as not to take life too seriously. She likes to explore different spiritual and religious beliefs and has dreams of one day travelling abroad and seeing more of the world.

AS I REMEMBER IT

Laura Asay-Bemis

With at least three nurses toiling with their particular tasks in this small room with little ventilation and no windows, I carefully stood onto an approximately one foot step stool and lifted myself onto a chilly stretcher covered with a mere sheet. Doctor Storm and Steve the Anesthesiologist entered the room. I felt like I had no control over what was about to happen. The doctor began placing probes on my head by firmly attaching silver dollar size electrode pads bilaterally. Chills went through my body. An elevating fear rose from deep inside me as I smelled the aroma of rubbing alcohol being placed on my temples. The scent churned my stomach and still to this day the stench of alcohol takes me back in time . . . a time I wish I could forget.

A private joke bantered back and forth between the nurses and Doctor Storm, as he said to his colleagues in a joking manner, "Did you hear what Doctor Jones said during the staff meeting about the new Psychiatrist having no voice except for the one in his head?" Everyone began to laugh but me. I felt alone, like a small child being dropped off in kindergarten with no friends, just strangers all around. This rapidly rising fear left my soul as I became numb to what was happening. Without anyone saying "hello" or "good morning" the commotion began.

One nurse began taking away my control by strapping my ankles and wrists down with restraints made of what felt like cotton with a bit of nylon mix. They were light beige in color. Another nurse strapped a tourniquet around my left upper arm then wiped it with alcohol, a familiar and triggering smell. She began to poke and prod through the massive quantity of IV scar tissue looking for a vein that would hold. Often scar tissue becomes very pronounced in a vein, after being stuck within the same area multiple times. Finally a usable vein was found and the IV hung.

A third nurse placed a blood pressure cuff on my right arm and one on my lower left leg just above the ankle. I felt pressure on my lower leg, but the restraints held me still. I could not see the turmoil going on around me as a strap was placed over my forehead holding me still.

Preparation went fast and then I heard Steve say in a calming voice, while placing a mask over my mouth and nose, "I want you to count backwards from 20." I complied with the request. At number 17 I awoke in the recovery room. Disorientated and dazed from the anesthesia I began to awaken and through blurred eyes, I saw other patients to both the right and left of me lying motionless. The smell of alcohol surrounding us all. I slowly looked down at my shirt and was jarred awake by the sight of blood splattered on the T-shirt, which was originally white. A nurse heard me gasp. She hurried over and said, "Don't worry. Your IV came loose during treatment and a bit of blood squirted out." Still in a fog, I drifted back to sleep. (When my IV had come loose during the brief seizure that is induced by the procedure, instead of IV fluid going in my arm, blood started to come out). Usually the IV is securely taped in place but mine had jarred loose.

It was my second of three Electroconvulsive Therapy (ECT), "shock," treatments that week. This procedure seems to change the brain chemistry helping with some mental illnesses. The 5-10 minute procedure is often used when medications and other types of therapy have shown to be ineffective.

On Mondays, Wednesdays, and Fridays my days seemed almost ritualistic; get up, get dressed, get in the passenger side of the car, be escorted by my mother to the local psychiatric hospital. I would enter the hospital in almost a comatose daze from all the heavy prescription medication I was given. While doing ECT, I was on three times the FDA recommended dose of an antidepressant and it was very sedating. ECT was recommended for my depression and suicidal tendencies as a last resort.

I was required to sign paperwork saying it was voluntary and of course a liability release. An intake nurse would say sign here, initial here, and even though my thoughts were a haze and I had no idea what I was doing, I complied with the request, and like a dead soul with no concern for life, I followed the instructions. All this paperwork would be done before the procedure. Following the paperwork, they told me I was being given a muscle relaxant shot in my upper hip and was sent back to the day room where I would find a couch or chair and do my best to recline. 'Good Morning America' played on the television lulling me to sleep. The muscle relaxant helped minimize the seizure that would soon be induced and helps further reduce injury.

I was told by Dr. Storm that a person will have two to three shock treatments weekly for 3 to 4 weeks totaling 12 treatments, (sometimes a few more). No one knows why or how ECT works to help severe mental illness, but many chemical aspects of the brain are changed during the seizure process. These changes build on each other and that is why a series of treatments are usually given for 4 weeks. However, I endured these treatments for 5 years and the procedures altered my memories, behaviors and life.

ECT works especially well for some individuals with few side effects. It's one of the fastest and most effective ways to relieve many of the symptoms of severely depressed or suicidal individuals. One of the symptoms can be memory loss. It is normal to lose some memory of the weeks or months before treatment, known as retrograde amnesia. This type of amnesia may or may not be permanent.

Unfortunately, I am one of the few people that ECT caused major memory loss. My short term and long term memory is damaged. I have very few childhood and young adult memories except for some traumas that held on. I rely on my friends to tell me about past pleasant experiences. My ECT took place in the mid-nineties when I was diagnosed with schizo-affective disorder and major depression. But that wasn't my first diagnosis, and it surely would not be my last.

I was first diagnosed as Borderline Personality Disorder, then Schizophrenia, which changed to Schizo-affective, then Post Traumatic Stress Disorder (PTSD), Seasonal Affective Disorder (SAD), Major Depression, Chronic Depression, Dysthymia. Now, I am being treated for Dissociative Identity Disorder (DID) also known as Multiple Personality Disorder, with Recurrent Depression.

I have Alters (Personalities), and some of those personalities lean towards different diagnoses. Perhaps that's why I have been diagnosed with so many conditions. DID is a severe form of dissociation where I lack a connection between my thoughts, feelings, actions, memory and sense of identity. DID affects about 1% of the population. The memory loss is due to having DID and ECT.

Along with memory loss, I have other mental illness symptoms. I hear internal voices, God talks to me, I have insomnia and I struggle with self-abuse and suicidal ideation. I have been in therapy since 1995 with a variety of therapists, psychiatrists and psychologists. Although I do not understand DID fully, I am learning about my diagnosis through therapy about the way my mind processes information.

I have also learned a significant amount about my family. I was raised with two sisters. Maggie was eight years older. The middle child, Sue, was 4 years older than I am. Maggie and Sue didn't get along, fought physically and yelled all the time. I never really knew much about Maggie, since by the time I was 9 years old she had moved out of the house and left Sue and I together. Sue was severely mentally ill and would physically hurt me, emotionally abuse me and yell at me. I was scared of my sister.

When Sue was 12 years old she ran away. While Sue was gone, I felt a sense of calmness. That peace lasted four years until she returned home. Living on the streets for four years, Sue came home even more psychologically challenged than when she left. Her diagnosis was manic-depressive or better known now as bi-polar. Maggie struggled most of her life with depression. She began having kids at an early age and throughout her life she had many boyfriends that fathered her children.

Both of my siblings relied financially and emotionally on my dad. Sue relocated to the same small town in Oregon that Maggie lived in, when I was in my first year of college. Both became dog groomers and worked in that small town constantly fighting for customers and fighting against one another. Sometimes they had restraining orders against one another.

Both my mother and father lost their battles to cancer. Sue and Maggie were devastated when dad died. Sue became very lonely and wanted a group of friends she could rely on. One day a religious organization came to Sue's house and befriended her. This organization explained that she must stop smoking cigarettes and could not do drugs or alcohol. Sue never drank alcohol, but was a two pack a day smoker and drank over a liter of diet coke. Sue tried to stop smoking immediately and stopped all her medications, since medications were drugs. She stopped the soda because caffeine is a drug. Surely, this would help her gain this religious organization's approval.

As a result of suddenly discontinuing her medication, Sue was rushed to the hospital from withdrawal symptoms. The doctors tried to give her medication, so she left the hospital against medical advice. Late that night she told me "Laura, I have put aside some things for you and some coins, I can't go to the hospital because they want to give me drugs and I can't have them." I told Sue I would come help her. I got the next flight to Oregon; but I did not make it in time. Sue chose to end her life three years after dad's death. Nine months after Sue died, Maggie's depression escalated out of control. I had no idea how depressed Maggie was until I got the call from my niece saying Maggie had taken her own life. That fast, my family was gone. Mental illness can have a genetic component and the Bemis family definitely has it.

After losing my family, I was lost in my thoughts and had to get involved in the community to persevere. I got involved in the National Alliance on Mental Illness (NAMI) by becoming a speaker, support group facilitator and instructor for various mental health programs. I enjoy my volunteer work with NAMI and spreading hope by sharing a variety of my life experiences showing that mental illness is not who you are, but it is a small part of your life story. I also tell some of my story for the Stop Stigma Sacramento: Mental Illness is Not Always What You Think campaign. I have so many traumatic memories and so few pleasant memories that telling bits of my life story is a reminder of how far I have come in my journey. I also hope that sharing my life, my family dynamics and my current state of mind, will help others see mental illness in a new light.

I graduated from California State University, Sacramento with a Bachelor's degree that I designed myself. Although my mental illness started when I was in my early 20's, I managed to "keep it hidden" until my late 20's. It is not uncommon to avoid seeking help for a mental health condition for many years due to the stigma and ignorance around mental illness. I finished college early, graduating with a Fine Arts and Photography B.A.

I keep very busy so I can stay present and not regress into past traumas. I have learned many coping tools and have been through various types of therapy and do mindfulness exercises. I know that if I don't work on my mental stability daily, I will fall back into an unhealthy lifestyle. I work part-time in the Mental Health and Substance Use Disorder field. Being a Consumer/Family Member Consultant, I run focus groups to assure individuals who receive Medi-Cal services have adequate care.

When I am not working part-time, or helping with NAMI and Stop Stigma Sacramento, I volunteer my services elsewhere. Some of my volunteer positions include being the Secretary of the Sacramento County Mental Health Board and the Founder of a Sacramento County funded Art Exhibit called Journey of Hope: Real Life Stories of Living with Mental Health Challenges Portrayed Through Art. And if that isn't enough, I am also a Professional Photographer with a mobile photography business. I enjoy teaching photography to adults and using the photographic arts to bring others a new way of viewing the world.

I came from a dark place in my life full of trauma, self-abuse and betrayal, to a place where I now consider myself successful and engaged in the community. With the help of a great support team made up of professionals and many friends, I thrive in spite of having a mental health condition. I have many skills that I have developed over the years and at the same time I have spent many a day in a psychiatric facility.

Success, for me, is not how much money I make or what my career choice is. Success is what you make it. For some it is getting out of bed. Success for me is putting one foot in front of another and continuing on the road to recovery. I know progress does not happen without a struggle. There is Hope for recovery and my mental health challenge is a journey and not a final destination. When life seems unbearable I remind myself, 'This Too Will Pass.'

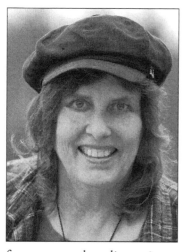

ABOUT LAURA ASAY-BEMIS

Laura is a professional photographer, a Consumer Representative on the Sacramento County Mental Health Board and a speaker for Stop Stigma Sacramento Speakers Bureau. She is very active in the National Alliance on Mental Illness (NAMI) as a certified speaker, support groups facilitator and Peer to Peer class instructor.

Laura also runs focus groups for an external quality review organization to assure Medi-Cal clients are receiving appropriate mental health and substance abuse services throughout California.

Laura uses her photographic skills to help in her own mental health recovery and teaches photography to others to allow them to see the world in a new way.

Although Laura lives with Dissociative Identity Disorder (DID), previously known as Multiple Personality Disorder, Complex Post Traumatic Stress Disorder(C-PTSD) and Depression, she works daily on her journey towards recovery. Laura has always been very active in her community with a positive attitude and tireless energy to encourage others to be the best they can be.

OUR STORY MATTERS

Rebecca Bakken

Sharing our truth, authentically with others is not easy, especially the pieces we deem dark and ugly. We fool ourselves into isolation, pulled in by our own narrow mindedness, brain lies, and limited perspectives. As children we celebrate princesses, superheroes, and happy endings. We are taught early on that our sorrows and struggles are to be shaken off, dismissed, fixed, or otherwise repressed. There are times, too, when we share with the wrong people or in the wrong manner. And when our expectations are not met, we often form resentments and retreat. However today, I know in my bones that there is deep wisdom in understanding how our personal traumatic events have caused trauma warping our thinking, behaviors, relationships and perspective.

I learned early on that sharing 'the truth' would not change my circumstances nor did it bring me comfort. As a survivor, I was simply trying to navigate everyday life and act 'normal'. So that is what I did . . . act, mimic, pretend, distort or all together disassociate from reality. My story was that my story did not matter.

I was born the second of four children. We lived secluded on a beautiful property in a small country town with lots of room to run and play. I fondly recall days filled with mud pies, tree forts, and tire swings. Once the sun went down it was anyone's guess how Dad would come home. Most likely, he'd be drunk or on drugs after stopping at the local bar on his way home. He may be the goofy drunk and making us dance with forced smiles and pounding hearts. Or maybe the super 'fun' and crazy drunk that wants to put me on the back of his motorcycle and take me for the ride of my life. Or our least favorite, psycho black-out drunk.

I was not the same fearful child at school that I was at home. When I stepped onto the bus it was like walking through a portal. As I got older, I was increasingly aware that I was another person outside of my home. In early childhood I was deemed overly sensitive, emotional, sad, and anxious. School was a haven from the chaos at home. I found it easy to make friends and teachers liked me. I adored my third-grade teacher. Each week she'd pick a student to receive "The Bucky Beaver" reward. This meant being the teacher's pet and other special privileges for the week. I could hardly wait, but the day never came. Mom had another plan in place. While we were at school, Dad went to work, and she went to the police with broken facial bones and her protruding black eye. She filed a report, restraining order and made plans for us to flee. She would finally accept that we were in imminent danger. First, we stayed briefly at a 'safe house,' followed by a hotel room until we went to stay with my grandparents. My Mom would have to fight for our custody and through an unbelievable turn of events my Father became the custodial parent of me and my younger brother and sister.

Without haste Dad met and married an eighteen-year-old woman. Her presence brought me comfort and a welcomed, but false, sense of safety. She cared for us, but the honeymoon was short lived. My dad's drugging and drinking was progressively worse. The violence continued. One terror I recall was watching her get pulled down a steep rocky hill, more than a hundred yards, face down, flailing about and bouncing off the ground. I have only a few clear recollections of the traumatic incidents that occurred, but this is one of them. She would be the second woman to flee from my father afraid for her life. This would also be the second time I was abandoned by my 'caretaker' and left behind. My dad was happy to keep the job as my custodial parent. Sometimes Dad would take me and my siblings to the roller-skating rink for an all-night skate and dance party. He would drop us off for the night, go to his own party, and pick us up in the morning. I loved going, hearing the loud music, dancing, cute boys, eating the snack bar food! It was heaven for a 'normal' thirteen-year-old. I used to drool over this older high school guy who had come every week. He would always dance with the prettiest girl there and one night I was the lucky one! We danced hot and heavy and later I agreed to sneak out of the rink and go for a night stroll. Maybe I will get my first kiss? His house was conveniently close to the rink. He invited me in. I got my first kiss and more. Within minutes he was pulling down my pants. I had no idea what was happening. He held me down and proceeded to rape me. That morning dad picked us up and I swallowed a bottle of Tylenol.

This would be the first sexual assault and my first attempt to take my life. There would later be a second assault, followed by a second attempted suicide. And a fucking third! I am hesitant to share, that I was not one that found comfort from the #MeToo movement, particularly some of the sharing and sensationalism on social media. As an empath it was triggering to hear the countless stories of other victims' experiences. It is my hope that we elevate the conversation to what happened to us, personally as the result of traumatic events. I am equally aware (and can empathize) with the brokenness of the perpetrators and our societal response to this dual sided tragedy of humanity. I find comfort and healing working within a therapeutic setting with experts that specialize in trauma. Finding the proper care was an arduous task but the relentless pursuit was not for nothing. Without my care team today, I could not even speak this truth to myself much less to You!

By 13 years old I had dissociated on a fundamental soul level. I did not experience life the same way again. I no longer prayed to God to save me from my life. Instead, I just faked living. I reflected to the world whatever they saw me as. At school I was an outgoing, well-adjusted kid: student government, cheerleader, athlete, good student, liked by most and hated by other pretty girls; check, check, check. During my sophomore year of high school Dad began to spiral down even further, drinking more and becoming increasingly abusive. I recall going to cheer camp at UCSC. Dad signed up to attend the trip as a chaperone (crazy, I know!) and the first night we were there he passed out cold outside of his hotel room. The other parent chaperones had to wake me to assist in getting him to bed. When my compartmentalized lives, home and school, collided I was devastated. He beat my sister and I for the last time when we did not clean our room well. I was hurt badly, but it was the vacancy in his eyes, looking at me but seeing right through me. It was our time to flee. At seventeen, just before entering my junior year, I called my mom and after a short time the three of us were in her custody. I did not transition well. I was a broken person and I found myself befriending other broken people. Somehow, I graduated high school and for the first time I began to contemplate the future. I jumped at the opportunity to move away with my oldest sister. Independence was fun and exciting, but it was clear that I was maladjusted to life and needed to seek therapy. So, I did. The first time I saw a doctor for my poor mental state I was prescribed Prozac. My reaction to this medication was not typical, but I have been told by psychiatrists that it likely triggered a bipolar episode resulting in mania and attempting suicide. I did not stop seeking help.

My efforts to find support doubled down when my Dad was arrested and convicted of murdering his third wife, Katherine. I do not know anything about the events that took place leading up to her death. I did not know this woman well, but I still carry sorrow for her loss. I pray for her mother and children. My father spent the rest of his days in prison and just passed in December of 2020. He loved his kids more than anything in the world! He was one of the most remarkable, talented, hardworking, kind people I have ever known. My dad had his own history of abuse, sexual assault, abandonment, and untreated mental disorders. He was already broken when I came on the scene. I miss him just as much today as I did the day I left.

At nineteen I stumbled upon a 12-step program to learn more about how to recover from a dysfunctional alcoholic upbringing. This would set me on a path toward healing that I could have never imagined in my wildest dreams. A dear friend, Shoshanna, referred me to Francis Weller (MFT, psychotherapist, writer, and soul activist). He helped bring me back to life. My eyes swell with gratitude just recalling the abundance of patience, compassion, and other gifts this man brought to my life. For years he worked tirelessly with me in the traditional behavioral therapy sense where I filled up my tool bag. His care and guidance opened me up to a world beyond self. I tended and mourned deep wounds. His quest to share deep soul healing restored my broken heart. For nearly ten years I was part of a community that transcended friendship. Together Michael, Kirk, Candy, Shoshanna, myself and many others learned together how to welcome our broken parts, find purpose, celebrate gratitude, and make life sacred not separately but collectively. The Universe opens when we live aligned with our heart and not compartmentalized. During this period, I experienced peace, purpose, gratitude, and home for the very first time.

By twenty-three I was moving right along checking new, more mature boxes: amazing supportive people in my life, good job, paying all my own bills, working two jobs, and attending junior college. Killing it! What's next? I had already had my fill of bad boys and I no longer wanted the chaos of a dysfunctional relationship. I met Eric and it was the first intimate relationship I had of true substance. He was not just compelled by my good looks and charms, he genuinely wanted to get to know me, my life story, and my heart. I wanted to gobble him up. I wanted him to spend all his time with me, adore me, and let me wear his t-shirts. But he liked himself, valued his personal time, liked his own t-shirts, and did not want to spend every second with me. He had a relationship with himself that I admired and I wanted this kind of self-love. Eric had a practice of expressing anger that I observed where we met working together. He would go out behind the building and take a sledgehammer to the side of the dumpster. This was to me an honest expression of frustration that he learned to exercise in a manner without consequence or damage to others. He tended to his feelings, got it out of his system and came back to the office ready to approach the circumstances from a fresh perspective and a smile. Man of my dreams; check. Bring on the babies!

At 29 I was pregnant with our first-born son. It was an incredibly empowering experience. I have never felt more grounded or strong as did while carrying, and later birthing him. When he was placed on my belly, he crawled up toward me with such astounding determination. He came with a purpose, and I knew it. Becoming a parent with all its joys and glories was soon foreshadowed by new boxes; endless obligations, responsibility, fear, unrealistic expectations of myself and my husband consequently. I was so obsessed with providing everything that I did not have that I ditched every anchor that prepared me for him! We quickly made a geographical change to be near family. I sought promotions and dollars to provide for my family and I worked like an ox all day and nursed my son to sleep for hours, literally for hours, every night for 18 months. I thought I was doing all the things. But what I did not see was that every day I was abandoning myself, health and values for self-imposed obligations. My sleep cycle was destroyed, and I began to rely on alcohol to relax and get to sleep. I wanted to buy him a house and provide him the best education possible and of course have a second child! Check, check, check.

My second pregnancy looked a lot different, and it was a direct reflection of my self-care. Kai Jason was born in 2009. He was an easy baby, full of laughter, curiosity and observant. With his arrival I internalized additional pressures that made my life unmanageable. While I continued trying, I was exhausted from sprinting and could not see a finish line. I was picking up more and more coping mechanisms that were self-destructive. In 2011 following the third assault I became a shell of a human being, hell bent on destroying myself, living in my failures, immersed in self-loathing and contempt. As a mother and wife taking my life was no longer an option. I knew that would cause irreparable damage. My bootstraps were my children and family. I could not fight for myself, but I had to for their sake. I had support from my husband, children, friends and extended family. I know that I am very lucky to get to say that.

It would be many long years, many wrong doctors and therapists, many wrong medications and a tireless effort on my part to finally learn how to advocate for myself within the many limits of our mental health care system. A year ago, I was diagnosed with Complex PTSD, Dissociative Disorder, Bipolar 2, and Alcoholism. With this diagnosis came medication that has changed my ability to meet life on its terms. For the first time ever, I can sleep peacefully, to pause my thoughts, and reel in emotional flooding. Medication has not been a cure-all for me. There are many ways I must hold myself accountable for my being and staying well. This includes a care team of specialists that have provided me the tools, resources, support, medication and competence that I needed to repair my broken, beautiful brain.

David Zuccolotto, PhD, clinical psychologist, author and former Pastor is currently my therapist. He has spent hours in session with me at the white board answering countless questions about brain functions. He introduced me to useful books* and then helped me digest and apply the things I learned. Once I understood some things about the brain intellectually, I was able to slowly accept the full scope of my pain and meet myself where I truly was, not where I wanted to be. I had to trust if we went into my psyche that I would come out alive. He demonstrated a care and caution that allowed me to begin to tell my truth. I headed his cautions and embraced his suggestions (most of the time). His background as a pastor lent a certain sacred quality to our therapy. It was his encouragement to build my own relationship with God that would catapult my rehabilitation.

Curtis Buzanski (LMFT, with an advanced certification in addiction counseling (LAADC) and trained in EMDR and The Comprehensive Resource Model) has helped me to understand the interplay of addiction and dual diagnosis. To date this has been the most effective form of trauma therapy. Our session begins with a phone call. This is important because I must know when my mind is off track in order to pick up the phone. I will try to articulate the actual process, but it is truly a modality that must be experienced. In a safe comfortable environment, a typical session begins by identifying a specific emotion attached to a triggering memory. After a brief check-in we begin using bi-lateral stimulation, relaxation and deep meditative breathing. I am able to fully inhabit my body while setting aside the ever protective (lying) brain. In this safe space I can access, hold, and find internal resources to repair the crippling emotions attached to traumatic memories. On the other side is a profound sense of clearing out the wreckage and new strength from within that I get to take out into the world.

My psychiatrist, Sufen Chiu, MD listened to me from the get-go (unlike many of her predecessors). I trust her competence as she monitors my symptoms and medications with care and keeps me chemically on track.

I have an amazing tribe of women that I cherish. We help keep one another sober by sharing our experience, strength and hope with each other. We come together when life gets hard, and we celebrate life's joys. With this unconditional support I have been able to repair and amplify my spirituality. My prayer used to be a single acronym- WTF? But today, I get to live a soul led spiritual life with God, nature and my people. I know I have only just begun to share this gift and help others uncover and rewrite their story.

ABOUT REBECCA BAKKEN

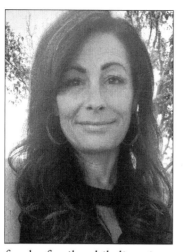

Rebecca and her family- husband Eric, and her sons Lucas and Kai- live in California near Sacramento. She currently enjoys her work as an independent startup consultant for small businesses and nonprofits. She's fortunate to have clients that appreciate her balance of passion, competence and results. Rebecca enjoys free time in the garden and being outside in nature. If not there, she's likely cooking gourmet food for the family while listening to funky music (hold the wine). At the forefront of her everyday life is service, joy, and wonder!

Reach Rebecca at:

Rebecca4change@gmail.com

HOW CONNECTION SAVED MY LIFE

David Bartley

Augu st 31st, 2011 was, by all appearances, just an average day. It was, in fact, a Wednesday, a "hump" day, not extraordinary in any way but one; this was the day I was going to kill myself.

This was the day the wretched monster known as clinical depression, after a close to a 40-year bloody fight, landed a fatal blow to my mind. That punch to my psyche finally convinced me what he had been telling me for years; I was weak, pitiful, stupid, and utterly grotesque and without merit or worth.

Now having me on the ropes, the monster switched to the role of "good cop," assuring me the pain of existence would end in the 7 ½ seconds it would take my body to fall 730 feet from the deck of the Foresthill Bridge. And the monster concluded by promising me that every single person in my life would be far better off once I was dead.

Those lies in hand, accepted by me as absolute truths, I walked out the front door of my home and into my Dodge Dakota pick-up truck, the one painted a bright emergency red.

I put the key in the ignition and turned it to the right. In an instant, the engine roared to life. But before putting the truck into gear, I took one last look around the beautiful 2 ½ acres of my property. After a moment, I took a deep breath, put the truck in gear, and without telling anyone where I was headed, I began the short 20 min drive to that tall, tall bridge.

It is essential to note that this was not the first time I had made this trip. My constant suicidal ideations had convinced me of the need to have the specifics of a plan readily available. Obedient to the command, I had made this trip many times, underscoring that killing oneself is rarely spontaneous.

Arriving at the bridge, I parked in the spot I had previously mapped out, turned off the motor, then reached over to the passenger seat and took hold of the suicide note I had typed out.

I placed the note in the center of the dash and then put the keys in the note's center. I exited the vehicle and then spun back around to make sure I had left the door unlocked.

I crossed the road, turned right, and headed down a narrow trail that ran parallel with the busy road. I walked 1,000 feet until I reached the mid-point of the bridge deck.

Once there, I turned to my left, and then pressed my body against a 4 ½ foot suicide barrier and completely stretched my arms to each side. Instead of looking out and taking in the spectacular view, I looked down to an oval-shaped spot of water in the middle of the North Fork of the American River that ran perpendicular to the bridge far below.

The river was swiftly flowing, but in my mind's eye, the water was stationary, not moving at all. The illusion became a target to focus on, a life-ending "bulls-eye."

In the next moment, I closed my eyes and began rehearsing the move up and over the barrier, imagining the speed of my fall and whispering aloud a prayer that somehow, I would die before I hit the water.

In that place of total fixation, to this day, I cannot tell you how long I remained hunched over the rail, peering down, teetering on my final movement. But, thankfully, it was long enough for a passing driver to look upon the scene, and realize, something's not right with this picture.

In turn, that soul called 911 and a 1st responder then approached me from the left-hand side and did two things. First, he established contact, which is logistical, and then he created a connection that is lifesaving because connection creates hope and hope saves lives.

I was taken off the bridge, then to the ER, and ultimately to a psychiatric hospital where I would remain for the next 15 lifesaving days.

But, when people found out I was in a locked-down psych ward, and why I was there, they were shocked. Those closest to me stood in the uneven space of utter confusion. They were perched there, frantic, and bewildered because instead of seeing me as clinically depressed and suicidal, people saw me as the happy and contented co-director of a larger, nationally recognized animal sanctuary.

The sanctuary was an extraordinary and sacred place. Our little slice of heaven was home to as many as 100 wonderful animals: 25 horses, 23 dogs, 9 potbelly pigs, umpteen sheep and goats, ducks and geese, bunnies, and birds, even an assortment of turtles and fish.

What made the sanctuary genuinely unique was that each animal fit into one of four categories; they were either very old, very sick, had some special needs, or were at the end of their lives. Because of this, we did no adoptions and became widely known as a "Forever Home" to those companion animals deemed "unadoptable." And on June 2, 2010, the sanctuary was featured as the cover story in the Life section of USA Today.

In no way did I fit the image of someone who was mentally ill, clinically depressed, or suicidal. But the truth is, sometimes what hurts the most can't be seen. Sometimes great despair and soul-wrenching agony lie just behind a forced smile, a distracting joke, or the façade of a seemingly perfect life.

Hiding my suffering behind the velocity of caring for animals in need, no one knew the depth of anguish I felt nor the true measure of hopelessness that had overtaken me. And just 14 months after the article appeared in USA Today, there I was with the hand of the monster in the middle of my back, nudging me ever closer to the point of no return.

But connection saved my life. I was convinced that August 31, 2011, would be my last day alive. Instead, it became the first day in a brand-new life, and the first steps in what has now been a 10-year journey, away from the frigid space of mental "hellness" and into the warmth and security of mental wellness.

A journey I continue to this day and will for the rest of my life.

ABOUT DAVID BARTLEY

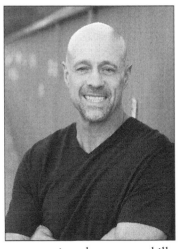

As a mental health speaker, educator, and advocate, David Woods Bartley has seen his fair share of successes and setbacks, from directing a nationally recognized nonprofit to battling a life-threatening mental illness. The latter was a brutal knock-down, drag-out fight with clinical depression that led David to a suicide attempt.

His life having been saved, David is committed to moving the conversation about mental illness and suicide from the dark shadows where they now live to the forefront of public concern. In doing so, David's mission is to transform the perception of mental illness from a life-threatening condition to that of a heroic cause, a level ground of understanding where those who suffer are no longer shunned but instead embraced.

Currently, David is a member of the NAMI, the International Association for Youth Mental Health, and the National Storytelling Network's Healing Story Alliance and holds certifications in Mental Health First Aid, SafeTALK, and QPR.

In addition to giving a TEDx talk and being named a 2021 Mental Health Champion by the Steinberg Institute, David has delivered more than 500 presentations on mental health, suicide, culture, and leadership to audiences across the United States, Canada, Central America, and India.

REMOVING THE MASK AND HEALING

Natalie Conrad

Running upstairs from the basement, her mind is spinning. She nearly trips as she reaches the landing. The tears cannot be held back any longer; she stifles her cry. Rushing into the bathroom, she shuts and locks the door quietly. "What can I do?" She thinks to herself. "My life is horrible. I can't ever be good enough, no one listens to me, and no one understands the pain I feel." Then, she has an idea—to end it. If her life was over, then she would not be haunted by this pain, the pain of living inside a "sweet, smart girl with proper manners" body where no one seems to hear, or care about, her cries for help. She opens the medicine cabinet and takes out a bottle of pills.

That desperate girl's name is Natalie. I am that girl and I took those pills and lay down, like Snow White, for a long peaceful sleep. Only I wasn't waiting for my prince to come. I wanted death. I wanted the horrible, deep pain to end.

I don't know how long I was out, but I do remember being angry that I woke up. Why didn't I die? I took a whole lot of pills. This is how my life goes—nothing goes the way it is supposed to. Now I have a secret, the first of many that I cannot tell anyone because they will see me as flawed. My family frowns on being real; they prefer perfect. They have an outer façade. My family of origin pretends they are happy, proper Southerners who go to church and help other poor souls in need. What about my poor soul?

After my suicide attempt at 13, nothing changed; I just "dealt" with it. By dealing with it, I mean I never shared what happened, until 39 years later. I tucked it underneath my heart and tried to forget. Haunting emotional pain was my constant companion and a hidden secret. Outwardly I continued to excel in all the areas important to my family—school, of course, but also in choir, drama and church. I spoke a second language, was a Girl Scout and seemed like I had a happy life. This was the beginning of what I call "wearing the mask." You know that kind of girl; I was grandma's favorite and the teacher's pet most of the time. Just think back to your days in school. Her name may have been Taylor or Alex instead of Natalie, but you know who I am talking about. She wasn't as popular as the cheerleaders or the jocks, but she was an A (if not straight A) student, who ran for student body office, dressed conservatively and you never once heard her swear.

For many years I blamed, I rationalized, and I kept up my façade. In my mind, my problems stemmed from my family. In fact, I blamed my family for 20+ years as the cause of my secret, horrible pain. Yet life goes on, and I did what everyone else was doing: I got married.

In my late 20's, as a mother of three, I was diagnosed with depression. I tried hard to overcome it and thought, quite a few times, that I had beaten it. I was prescribed medication, which I took but never spoke about. I read all the self-help books on codependency, being a stronger person, and how to be successful. I saw a therapist and did a 12 step program for depression. I was trying to heal, to *get over* the depression. At one point I took myself off my medication. That didn't work; I became suicidal again. So I went back to the doctor, was assigned a psychiatrist by my medical plan and was put on not one, but two different pills that time.

There were many adjustments to my medication dosages in the beginning, and I was eager to be healed. The psychiatrist warned me that I was not to take myself off the medication because the suicidal thoughts could come back if I did so. In the meantime, my marriage fell apart for a variety of reasons; mistakes made by my husband and me. He didn't understand depression and, come to think of it, I really didn't either.

At 30 years old I was a single mom, working full time, taking my kids to daycare and my daughter to therapy, as she was diagnosed as being developmentally delayed. I was doing okay, all things considered . . . Then I met this guy and started to date. After an unexpected whirlwind of getting engaged and changing jobs, we decided to move in together. Now there were five children, not three, and we were adjusting. Or at least I told myself that we were all doing great.

But slowly things in my world, in my own mind actually, started to disintegrate. My new job was not going well, we were planning a wedding and looking at houses to buy. I got more and more weary each day, like I was coming down with the flu. I had to take naps when I got home before I could make dinner or check homework. My mind blanked frequently. I constantly forgot how I got to a destination even though I was the one driving. I couldn't seem to remember what I was going to say. And then one day, driving home on those same streets I had always taken, I saw a large redwood tree. I was in horrible pain inside my own head, and I found myself hyper-focusing on that tree. I told myself to grip the wheel, lock my elbows and accelerate. I could see the tree straight ahead. My head was spinning, and I was going to hit the tree. Then my thoughts hurled into an imagined future . . . a future without me . . . I thought about my kids . . .

I didn't drive straight into the redwood tree. Instead, I went home and got in bed to take a nap. This nap was different from other naps; I didn't get up to make dinner, I didn't check homework. I stayed in bed because I could not get up. This was not being lazy; it was about mentally not having the power to move my own body. Even though I did not kill myself, I was dead inside now—void of all feeling. I couldn't feel pain, love, or even the weariness I had felt in the days before. It was more than a numbness, this kind of absence of feeling. It felt as if I could not will myself to even exist.

After staying in bed for too many days, my fiancé sought help for me. I don't remember what happened, whom he called, where we went or how long it took, because I could not feel or recall anything.

The next thing I remember I was being admitted into a psychiatric center. There were beds, tables, chairs, and someone standing guard at the exit doors. I spent a week there trying to come back . . . back to life, back to my family, back to myself. My medications were adjusted again, and I saw a therapist every day and went to group therapy sessions. It felt as if I was trying to walk through a dense, heavy bog. There was resistance to every movement, and I became easily exhausted.

When I was released from the psychiatric center, I was still not whole. There were long naps several times each day, and I remember really trying to be "normal" when the kids got home from school so they would not worry—or worse yet, ask me more questions. There were many therapy appointments as well as lots of nightmares. I was instructed by my therapist to keep a journal.

A journal entry

This is the beginning . . . of many things—my recovery from depression, my discovery of inner self. It is the beginning of taking care of myself. My goal this week is to inspect my emotions. To look for keys, triggers . . . To feel some of the emotions [again] [and] not using the escape mechanism . . . These thoughts and feelings will no longer be a negative in my life - I am scared.

My recovery was a very slow process, and there was no rushing it. In fact, 20+ years later my recovery is still on-going. It is a journey that never ends. There have been some great scenery and memories along the way and some scary scenes and bad moments too. I have come to accept this. I have become more aware . . . aware of my feelings, aware of my need for support, aware of my triggers. I am living not just with my depression but in spite of it! I am always working hard to make the best of my journey. I see a therapist now on an "as needed" basis, and I am not afraid to tell others to seek therapy; it really does help.

As I head toward my 60s, my journey continues to take me to new places, physically, emotionally and spiritually . . . places I never thought I would go. You see, I have come to realize that many of the women in my family have suffered from depression or other mental illnesses. It has always been whispered about (never truly acknowledged), but has always been in the shadows. So many of them are wearing the mask too.

Now I acknowledge my depression. I began telling people my story in 2017. I am still a bit awkward when I start to talk about it and only do so when I intuitively know it is safe. Do you know what happens every time I talk about my mental illness? I find out that the person I am talking with is living with depression, is a suicide survivor like me, or has a family member or close friend with a similar story! He or she seems relieved to hear me talking freely about it. I now know that talking about mental illness helps normalize it, helps us all take off our masks, stops the whispers, lessens the shame, and begins to help others. I believe talking and educating others about mental illness lessens the stigma in our society.

Depression is a mental illness. It cannot always be seen when you look at a person. It is different for everyone; it lurks below the surface, wears that mask of normalcy, and yet the suffering is intense. There is help for depression and other mental illnesses, but the age-old stigmas that shamed the women in my family into silence are still pervasive today. Now is the time to talk openly about mental illness *and* mental health. Talking about depression can save a life from suicide.

Like everyone else, the older I get, the faster the years seem to fly by. All of our children are grown, and we have six grandchildren now. I belong to a fiber guild and enjoy many of the fiber arts. Most recently, I am learning to weave. After running my own business for 14 years, I am now working for a nonprofit that supports mental health organizations run by others with mental health diagnoses; we refer to ourselves as "Peers." I work with my fellow Peers in trying to fight for the rights of those who, like us, have a mental illness and want to live a productive life. A popular slogan we use is "Nothing about us without us." We advocate with policy and law makers and embrace diversity.

I have created a local nonprofit project called "Erase the Stigma Now," because I see firsthand how many things in society need to change to embrace mental illness as a condition as normal as physical illness. I have chosen to focus my efforts on stigma because, in my opinion, it is the first barrier.

Today I am an advocate and speaker who seeks to educate the mentally well about the stigmas perpetuated against those with a mental illness. When, as a society, we stop using words like "crazy," "cray cray" and "insane" to describe everyday occurrences, we help reduce stigma. Words can disrespect or minimize something that is very real and (very damaging) to someone within earshot of the conversations. The power of words can also heal. Mental illness is no one's fault! Eliminating stigma starts with knowing how to watch your language and how to speak about mental illness. Next, becoming educated on the warning signs of mental illness and how to respond will help you offer someone the right support without judgment.

Let's all begin to heal.

ABOUT NATALIE CONRAD

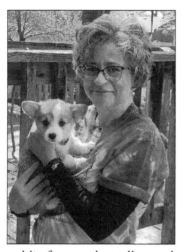

Natalie is an award-winning speaker and professional organizer who left her career field after she "came out" with her story of having a mental illness. She felt such relief in not living the lie of being "normal" that she began advocating for others who have been hiding their condition and pain due to the stigma of mental illness. Her nonprofit project is called Erase the Stigma Now. The project provides education and public forums that talk openly about mental illness and stigma. For more information or to help champion her cause, please visit www. EraseTheStigmaNow.org.

EVERYDAY MENTAL HEALTH

Joanna Dorman-Blackstock

My last and final bout of depression started after some divorce/custody related legal issues were finally resolved. After nearly three years of that challenge my fight, flight and even freeze instincts were fried. Adrenal fatigue, depression and now my new friend, anxiety, just weren't shaking off like I'd previously experienced. The beginning of the pandemic and shut down of the world made it even worse.

Just getting the basics was hard. I'd rather go back to sleep than get up to eat, drink water or even go to the bathroom. When I finally did muster up the energy, I'd do whatever work was needed for my job then back to the couch or bed. I had other bouts before, but something always forced me to keep going; kids, work, family and basic needs could only be put off for so long . . . unless there's a pandemic, then all bets are off. No office to go to, no lunch appointment with an optional healthy menu choice, no kids to take to school or happy hour to pop by (or get dragged to by well-meaning friends), absolutely nothing to propel me from the couch or out of bed. This time I was really scared. I'd lost my old driven, focused and resilient self for good. I wasn't ever suicidal, but my "give-a-flip" factor was negative 10,000 feet.

I had a few friends that would call for a walk along the river which was right outside my front door. If I had to drive to a location for an outing it was pretty much a no go.

Out of the blue a friend asked me to come to Las Vegas and help take his business from live events to an online platform now that the conference world was stalled for an unknown stint. It sounded like a nearly impossible feat, but something inside me knew I was spiraling into a place I didn't want to be or stay in for however many weeks the world would be closed. The promise of better weather was enough for me to be on a plane in less than 48 hours. That's when the discovery began. The change of scenery, patterns, and the removal of unhealthy options I'd previously been choosing to cope were eliminated by altering my environment.

We joked about it being my rehab, but that's ultimately what happened. First came a regular sleep schedule. Asleep by 10 pm and up at sunrise. At first light I was propped up on the patio facing the sun with a cup of tea until I was inspired to make a healthy breakfast. Sometimes that took 10 minutes and would take me over an hour on other mornings. Next, a little work and mid-morning exercise. There was no choice of unhealthy food since groceries were delivered from the market and I didn't make the grocery list in the beginning. After lunch, a little more work, then a 3-5 mile daily walk with the dog. Dinner happened every evening by 6-6:30 pm. We watched a little low engagement Netflix, then shower, to bed and repeat. This went on for 30 days. Developing this new routine of healthy habits allowed me to reset my whole nervous system. Within the first few days I stopped taking my antidepressants. I'm not suggesting anyone stop their meds without a doctor's supervision, but I had to do something. I was in a safe place with a controlled environment and a desperate desire to feel better. For me the meds made me feel worse. I was more tired, had less energy and felt completely unable to control my drive or focus on topics at hand. After 3 or 4 days I felt like a new person. I was mad and sad recognizing that this crutch that was supposed to be helping me revive my best self was actually taking me deeper into my demise.

I walked miles per day listening to books, podcasts, motivating orators searching for the right thing to make me feel better and more like my productive self. This is when I came across the work of Martin Siegleman. Otherwise known as the father of positive psychology, he explains the difference between cosmetic and curative medicines as they relate to antidepressants in his book *Flourish*. Antidepressants are cosmetic medicine. They only treat the symptoms and never cure the illness. Curative medication is like a shot of antibiotics to treat an infection. First light bulb, this medicine isn't going to cure my condition.

Seigleman spent decades as a therapist trying to help people overcome depression and other damaging mental illnesses before he transitioned into studying what made people happy. Another lightbulb, instead of focusing on how not to be depressed I needed to focus and expand on what made me happy at varying levels. Once my body chemistry was leveled out by eating properly, sleeping on a schedule, getting natural vitamin D and sufficient water anything was possible.

It seemed too simple to be the solution. I believe 100% that we can avoid slipping into a major depression or pull out of one by implementing these things. We know fresh air, healthy food and exercise are good for us. I didn't understand that by not committing to them in my lifestyle I was harming myself in ways I would never do intentionally any more than I would take illicit drugs or drive intoxicated.

For the last year I've continued to place a high priority on these basics. I don't get it right all the time, every week or every day. When I start feeling unusually fatigued, sluggish, apathetic or disinterested I look at these elements and typically something is off.

Guided meditation, a gratitude journal, supplements, humor and social connection are extensions for me in monitoring my everyday mental health now as well. Those are secondary to the basics of getting consistent quality rest, natural sunlight, proper nourishment, clean water and physical activity. Starting with just one of these elements at a time and habit stacking the others every few days will put you on the right path of controlling your everyday mental health. These are simple solutions, but have grace with yourself because it's not always easy . . . and that's ok. Just start by one lap around the block, a glass of clean water, sit in the sun or eat one healthy thing you enjoy. Do it again the next day and the next and then put a couple of those activities together. Before you know it you've built a foundation that's steady and stable.

ABOUT JOANNA BLACKSTOCK

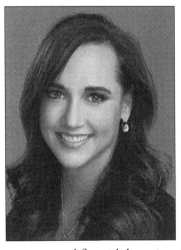

Real Estate Guru, International speaker/trainer/coach, Adventurer, Mom and Philanthropist.

JoAnna is recognized among the top 1% of real estate professionals in the U.S. currently serving as CEO of Keller Williams Green Meadow in Oklahoma. She is an international speaker, trainer, coach and writer with a driving desire to see individuals discover their passions and flourish by using their gifts in the world. In addition to her full time real estate career she coaches other professionals inside and outside of the real estate arena on how to maximize their performance while creating a personal lifestyle that compliments their biggest passions. JoAnna is the creator of the Soul Sparkle Jewelry Collection in collaboration with Soul Sparkle Living founder Hayley Hines. These designs are produced by women in developing countries to create economic growth opportunities that change their lives and affect decades to follow.

Awards/certifications:

- Certified Jack Canfield Trainer
- International Speaker on Women empowerment, emerging leaders & entrepreneurs
- Certified Floyd Wickman Trainer
- Top 25 Emerging Leaders in Tulsa
- 40 under 40 award by Tulsa Business Journal & Oklahoma Magazine
- Past President Women's Council of Realtors
- Board Member Tulsa Foundation for Architecture
- National Productivity Coach for realtors
- Team leader/CEO Keller Williams Green Meadow

FROM LOSS TO LOVE, LIGHT, AND LIFE

Cathleen Elle

When you tell people what you do for a living, what is the usual response? Perhaps they smile and nod in understanding because your job title says it all. Perhaps they look impressed with your accomplishments in a field that is a mystery to them, but that they recognize as respectable and important. Perhaps they silently thank their lucky stars that you do what you do so that *they* don't have to.

For me, sharing my job description generally also entails sharing a bit of my story—because when you say that you are, among other things, a "loss and grief expert," people want to know how you came to be an authority on those subjects. And so they hear that my son, Logan, took his life in 2010, and that I have since made it my mission to guide others through the pain associated with loss and trauma while also serving as an advocate for suicide prevention. Almost without exception, this brief explanation of my work is met with appreciation . . . and with some degree of sorrow or pity.

I can't blame people for reacting in this way. Losing a loved one is sad no matter what the circumstances. It may seem especially so when that loss is sudden and unexpected, and when the cause is extreme. But today, I'd like to share the side of my story that is occasionally overshadowed by its own tragic nature. I'd like to tell you what happens after the dust of a life shattered by loss settles, and the shell of a person sitting in the middle of it begins to rebuild from within. I'd like to show you, through my own experience, that whatever hardship you are facing now or will face in the future does not have to be a lethal blow; that you can create a new narrative around it; and that you can do more than just survive. You can thrive.

I should start with the tragedy itself, which struck when I was at the height of a 25-year career in politics. I had served four terms as a Vermont Legislator and had worked directly for the governor before taking on the role of executive vice president for one of the leading trade associations in the state. I was successful, I was well-known and well-respected, and I was confident in the trajectory of my professional life.

As for my personal world . . . That was a different matter. In the years leading up to Logan's passing, I was well aware that he was struggling internally, and we had seen numerous doctors who made different diagnoses and prescribed various medications to try to "fix" him, whatever that meant. I thought that I was doing my best for him—for both of us and for our family. I was an action-taker, a problem-solver, a changemaker who had accomplished more in my chosen field without any experience or college education than many of my more traditionally qualified peers. Surely I could figure out how to help my 19-year-old son through what I imagined we would someday remember as just a particularly rough patch.

Looking back, I know that I was, indeed, doing the best I could, given the knowledge I had at the time. I would come to question this assumption after he ended his life, however, because the unsuccessful treatment process had eaten away at our relationship to the extent that we hadn't spoken in several weeks before that fatal day.

The instant I found out, everything around me and inside

of me simultaneously froze and melted, a sensation that would rewind and repeat for months and years thereafter. Fear of and disbelief in something that had already happened mingled with guilt, shame, and pain. I should have done more. I could have solved this. But I had failed.

Ironically, the purpose that I eventually discovered—the purpose toward which I believe Logan himself guided me—manifested as almost a punishment at first.

During an especially low moment some four months after his passing, while I was lying and crying on his grave, the message that I was meant to do something with this tragedy, with my grief, with my son's story, came as clearly into my mind as if someone had spoken it. My body and soul must have been chomping at the bit for just such an assignment because I needed no other prompting. That very day, I set to work, allowing my natural drive and resourcefulness to lead the way. I made arrangements to assist the Vermont chapter of the American Foundation for Suicide Prevention (AFSP) with an upcoming annual fundraiser, leveraging the media connections I had developed over the course of my career to draw attention to the event, and ultimately raising over $13,000 through my efforts.

To this day, I can't tell you how many TV appearances I made, radio interviews I took, and newspaper articles I inspired. I only know that each one chipped away at my entire being, inevitably leaving me in tears or unable to function for hours afterward. By the time it was all over, I was physically and mentally drained from having continually recounted the collapse of my world, and—though I was proud of what I had done and grateful that I had been able to do it—I felt more guilt, more shame, and more self-hatred than I had when I began.

Why? Because in striving to raise awareness about the causes of and warning signs surrounding suicide, I was becoming more aware of those causes and warning signs, too. Each new tidbit of information I took in could be turned into a weapon against myself—a piercing confirmation of my negligence as a mother and my failure to recognize the numerous red flags that had been waving ominously around Logan for who knows how long prior to his final hours.

Self-isolation, withdrawal from activities, lack of motivation, erratic behavior, irritability and aggression toward loved ones, increased substance use . . . I had seen it all. And I had been too ignorant to take proper action. I was, as I had long suspected, to blame for Logan's premature exit from this earth. These were the self-judgmental, unforgiving, and unjustified messages that flooded my mind throughout that period.

In retrospect, I realize that, by diving so zealously into the fundraiser, I was attempting to erase those negative, accusatory feelings; to avoid my pain; to succeed in saving other people's lives where I had failed in saving my son's. And I had achieved a sort of success. But in doing so, I had left my "self"—the health of my body and mind—behind. I had reached another breaking point (the first having been the loss of Logan), and it was time for me to start picking up the pieces. It was time for me to heal.

If one thing had become clear to me over the course of those muddy months between Logan's passing and the conclusion of what I must have regarded as my rescue mission for lost souls at risk of suicide, it was that I needed help where my own well-being was concerned. It wasn't just that I couldn't bear the thought of looking too far inward, of uncovering whatever monsters I assumed were lurking in the darkest corners of my mind. I actually felt incapable of it. I didn't know how or where to begin, and there was still a very vocal part of me questioning whether or not I even deserved to try.

Yet some fighting spirit deep inside me, some instinct for survival, told my feet to do the walking and my mouth to do the talking while the rest of me followed along. And that's how I met Brooke, the cognitive behavioral therapist with whom I ended up working for years and who motivated me to seek many other indispensable resources, from support groups to mediums and everything in between. Words cannot express how grateful I am for the critical role she played in helping me to heal not only through the indescribable agony of losing Logan, but also through a host of traumas that my psyche had been hiding from me since my early childhood. With her gentle hand on my shoulder, I began the slow, illogical, back-and-forth journey of becoming whole again—or to put it more accurately, of becoming *new*, because I don't believe that any one of us is ever broken beyond repair.

No matter what horrors or sorrows we have experienced, no matter how fractured we may sometimes feel, all of our pieces are still with us; they are still ours. We simply need to decide that we are going to pick them up and, by combining them with the gifts we are given when we choose to care for ourselves—the gifts of self-knowledge, self-understanding, and self-acceptance—to build our present around our past, embracing it in the warm glow of healing.

Perhaps the most beautiful thing about investing in ourselves in this way is that the process, the progress, fuels itself. Once I made the choice to value and nurture my health, I actually grew interested in it. I *wanted* to learn what a body and mind—what *my* body and mind—needed in order to make it beyond a state of mere existence into a state of flourishing and even joy. Some of the tools I collected were incredibly basic, yet no less impactful for their simplicity. Eating well, getting enough sleep, spending time in nature, meditating, cultivating meaningful relationships with those who had stuck with me through the most difficult moments . . . These were all pretty straightforward changes for which I gradually carved out space in my routine.

At a certain point, however, I found that I wanted even more, and not just for myself; I wanted more so that I could share it with others. I wanted to find a way to turn our story—mine and Logan's—into a source of solace for anyone suffering from pain so consuming that it has the power to end a life and to ravage those with which it is intertwined. Somewhere along my path to peace, I had found my heart's calling—or rather, it had found me.

Through my work with energy healers, spiritual coaches, and mediums, and through my subsequent work *as* all of those things, I have gained so much: a fresh perspective on our inner worlds and just how expansive they can become; an understanding of the shift from life to death as a transition of energy rather than a full-stop ending; a certainty that those we have lost are forever with us, and that we are all capable of connecting with them if we open our spirits to the possibility . . . I could go on.

The most important lesson I've learned, however, is just how much I have to give—not in spite of, but because of all that I have experienced. And it is this that I offer to you. Whoever you are, wherever you are, you have my faith that, by choosing to step into your healing journey, you will survive whatever challenges you are facing; that you will evolve and expand through them; and that, with the self-awareness and acceptance you achieve, you will create a life of joy, light, and fulfillment.

ABOUT CATHLEEN ELLE

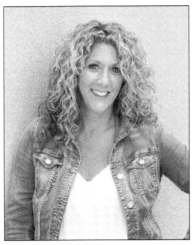

Cathleen is a transformational speaker, certified intuitive success coach, master healer, loss expert, author, and podcast co-host. By assisting people to move through layers of pain and trauma, and to break limiting beliefs, she revolutionizes lives. Her award-winning book, *Shattered Together: A Mother's Journey From Grief to Belief*—equal parts inspirational memoir and practical guide for those struggling with loss of any kind—is a #1 international bestseller on Amazon.

For more than twenty-five years, Cathleen served as a political leader in Vermont, working alongside the governor and as an elected legislator. She also lobbied for and led the Associated General Contractors of Vermont as executive vice president for nine years.

In March 2010, Cathleen's world was refocused when she lost her son to suicide. Through that shattering experience, she uncovered a powerful sense of self and a connection to the divine that motivated her to redesign her life—and to guide others in doing the same.

Today, Cathleen works with individuals who are interested in releasing the hold of past trauma, igniting the light within, uniting the head with the heart, and realizing their unique purpose. She is a certified success coach and a master energy healer specializing in Regenerating Images in Memory (RIM), a multi-sensory technique that facilitates mental, physical, and spiritual transformation.

In addition to providing personalized one-on-one assistance, Cathleen educates and inspires through public speaking engagements centered on suicide prevention, grief, self-discovery, and more at high schools, colleges, businesses, professional symposia, and a wide variety of other locations and events. She is also available for workshops, retreats, and creative partnerships.

As a collaborator, Cathleen has contributed to two inspirational anthologies, and she is a co-host of the weekly Beyond Your Best Plan podcast. She currently resides near her daughter in Charlotte, North Carolina, with two exceptionally enlightened cats.

To learn more on how to work with me or book me as a speaker, please connect with me:

https://cathleenelle.com/
FB Business Page: @cathleenelleinspires
FB Page: @cathleeninspires
IG: @cathleenelleinspires
Twitter: @cathleenelle
LinkedIn: @cathleenelleinspires

HOPE

Henry Johnstone

HOPE:

"A feeling of expectation and desire for a particular thing to happen, also a feeling of trust."

Hope can find its way into every fabric of our lives, and perhaps most poignantly it will find its way into the lives of those who need it the most, because hope is deeply understood by those who experience its darker side. Hopelessness.

I've written this so that someone else who is experiencing hopelessness might read this and know that all is not lost. No matter how dimly the light inside you flickers. There is hope, there is always hope. If you are beset by hopelessness you are one step closer to coming out of the other side.

I've had a mental health illness for as long I can remember.

From the first depersonalization episode at 11, through to emergent bi-polar, OCD, ADHD, anxiety disorder, dyspraxia and dyslexia. Although the last two are not strictly under the same banner they both added to the pot of what I used to think made me feel cursed. I found it hard to learn and to remember. Episodes of depersonalization left me shaking and terrified that

I was a stranger in my own head and my memories belonged to someone else. I felt frozen in the absence of self.

Now I believe them to be a blessing, a way to help build communities and an understanding of the suffering others experience on a profound level.

I want to share with you a memory from the dark days. It was the moment that in hindsight seems so utterly unlikely to have been a shift, but the more I have shared it, the more I realize it was.

In 2004 things were bad, as they say in AA, I was in the 'madness.' My mind was shredded and my body not far behind. Addiction spurring on and compounding an undiagnosed mental illness, which had me in a choke hold.

After years of stealing, lying, hurting and damaging my family I felt so agonizingly guilty and ashamed that I had left their house determined to suffer, like I needed to suffer. I felt wrong. My moods swung violently from sweetness and regret to blind rage and anger through to the pits of nothingness and profound meaninglessness, an absence of self. OCD meant I couldn't perform simple tasks without repeating them for hours or biting my skin and tongue in long periods of self-harm that leave me unable to speak. I was depressed, lost, violent. I was angry and I wanted to die in the most painful way possible.

The only time things made sense was when I was high, or drunk, or coming out of a self-harm episode. When I suffered it all made sense. So that's what I did, I made myself suffer. I welcomed every episode as further evidence that I deserved to feel this way.

I didn't know then what I know now. I wasn't a bad child, I wasn't a fuck up. I was in pain and I needed something to believe in, I needed some help. I had to trust again that I wasn't alone and that I deserved a life. But first I needed to admit that I needed help.

It was winter in Manchester, and early morning. I had been

woken up and moved on by police officers for sleeping behind a bus stop. I liked bus stops, there's a light directed away from the rear glass so whoever was there wouldn't be able to see me. I hated being seen. I hated the thought that they would see me. Not only physically see me, but see what I tried to blot out with drugs and drink. A child who was ashamed, lost and scared and a child who, despite all the shit they had done and the pain they had created, still missed his mum and wanted nothing more than to ask for forgiveness and ask for a hug.

I guess that was too painful for me to embrace. I didn't deserve it so I just put myself in positions that I thought were begetting of me.

I remember it being cold and experiencing some kind of loose pride that, as I had slept, the frost had laid over me. If it caused me damage then it was good for me.

I didn't set a course to where I ended up, it just happened. Through the walk there, I had sobered up and with no more booze in my system, that part of me that I had tried so hard for months to shut out came flickering back to life. I hated it so much. It had everything that I had tried so hard to avoid having. Feelings. Feelings were bad because feeling meant love, and love was not a feeling I could bare to feel. Love was connection and connection meant hope, and hope meant some life that was different from this one. That was too far to go. That was impossible. Maybe I'd walked here on purpose I don't know. I found myself at my parents' house. It was dark and no lights were on. I presumed my mother and father were asleep. I still have dreams of that house. They had a new door, I had kicked the other through after a frenzied drive to steal money, all so I could avoid that flickering light. I wasn't here to destroy anything, not tonight.

I wish I could tell you more about my feelings at this moment or why I did what I did and how I ended up as an emaciated boy crawling through a tiny basement window, glass sticking into my skin.

But I don't know why I chose to. I lay on the cold concrete floor, shivering and seeing my breath fog. I lay down and pulled my knees to my chest and I cried. Deep primal sobbing, my body shook and I let it. I cried to my mum. I cried to the feeling of her hugging me, the smell of her clothes, the perfume that in boarding school years past I had sprayed on a cloth to smell when homesickness struck. I was crying not to damage or suffer, I was crying to heal.

I hoped somewhere deep inside that three floors above me as she lay awake wracked with worry, my Mother felt something, a connection.

I don't remember how long I stayed there curled up on the floor. As the sun started to rise, I crawled out of the same window and left.

Something changed after that moment. I'm not going to lie and tell you that everything came together in the days that followed, because it didn't. I was still a child, and I was still lost but I had begun the shift toward a better life. By crying I had begun to face what I had long feared and pushed myself into darkness to avoid. This began to shift.

It was hope, and hope is difficult to contend with. We feel we are undeserving or we are so lost that there seems no way out other than a way which is infused with more suffering. Hope means that we are worth more than what we feel now, hope means that on some level we will have to accept that we are able to change and that it's going to be okay. I want you to know that I fought against hope so violently and destructively, I tried to murder all the hope that flickered inside me. I never thought that my life would change, much less so that I would be the one to change it.

My hope came from admitting all the feelings of pain I had harbored and kept locked away. Soon after, I began to reach out and build a network of people who understood me. I managed to build a bridge with my mother and in time I told her that I needed help, that I couldn't do this on my own. I went to rehab and got clean. I saw a therapist who helped me understand my emotions and work on the guilt and shame.

I began to forgive myself and slowly began to see life as filled with possibility. I found my greatest ally in psychotherapy. Here was a space where I could speak openly and gradually allow myself to be heard. The guilt, the shame, the paranoia, even the feelings of injustice and powerlessness. I wasn't judged. And within that I could begin to release the pressure cooker of emotions that had been building up for over 10 years. Not only that but this self-expression allowed me to explore the roots and triggers for my mental state. So often in mental illness we can feel at the mercy of our symptoms. Through therapy I learned about myself, why I respond to certain situations in certain ways. I began to heal because I understood myself and, in time, I would begin to cherish myself. Especially the wounded beautiful parts that I had tried too hard to hide. I attended rehab for my alcoholism and drug addiction. I worked hard to uncover and expose all my demons, to face them and heal them. Behind every trauma I learned there was a scared little boy in need of love. Addiction is disconnection so I did everything I could to connect to myself. It was amazing how the therapy I had was being tested, I paid £5 a session and it was transformative. My rehab was state funded and it was transformative. So often therapy and support is hidden behind a perceived pay wall. It has an exclusive feel to it. Every profession has the obligation to offer mental health support for free or for a vastly reduced cost.

I learned how to manage de-personalization. I allowed myself to experience depression. I learned ways in which to manage my ADHD and OCD. The dyspraxia still makes me very clumsy and my dyslexia still makes numbers unintelligible. Life is doable now where before it was not. My depression, anxiety, and OCD still surface from time to time. And that's okay, it's okay to not be okay. I am not infallible. I have my bad days. Now instead of being overwhelmed I have a tool kit for speeding along my recovery from an episode. Number one is community, a support circle, a group of people that can be told when an episode strikes. This is sharing and in that a connection is built so that I, and indeed you, don't have to do it alone. No one needs to suffer in silence and the simple act of sharing where you are and how you are, without the person trying to fix you, is so incredibly powerful.

I now consider myself as having turned my life around. I am in my 11th year (12 this April) of being clean and sober. I have found a good mix of medication to keep me level. I now work as a rapid change therapist using hypnotherapy and psychotherapy together to create shifts in emotional blocks and trauma from a subconscious level. The work is profound and from my own experiences I am able to understand the heartbreak and isolation from life. This is what I was born to do. I work with humble gratitude that I can be a port in the storm, (if you'll forgive the analogy) so that my clients can build a new boat and sail with freedom and excitement onwards.

There is a stigma that surrounds mental health, and it isolates those who need the care and support the most. We are at the cusp of change, a rewriting of the book on mental health, treatment, support, education and community. All of these must come together to initiate the kind of change that's needed. I implore you all to be a beacon of hope to anyone who is suffering, in recovery, or coping with mental illness from a child, friend, sibling or parent.

Our journeys mean we have to pass through periods of agonizing hopelessness and it is a journey that remains one of the most painful in human existence. Hopelessness cannot exist without it transforming into hope, and it is there for you. It has always been there for you and it always will be there. You are going to be okay, you are not alone, we are here for you.

ABOUT HENRY JOHNSTONE

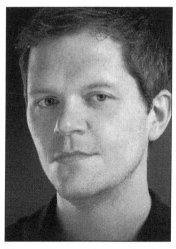

Rapid change therapist/Speaker/ Metalwork Artist

Henry is an unshakeable believer in the power of self. He is a driven and passionate voice for positive mental health. Henry's firm beliefs and hope for the future were born from hopelessness and adversity from a very young age. After 10 years of struggle with alcohol, drugs, and his mental health. Henry found himself in the hospital with a choice; carry on or change. Henry chose to change and has spent over a decade developing his mindset and approach to full recovery. Now aged 40, he has been clean for 12 years, he has turned his life around. Henry knows that nothing separates us more than the belief that we are different. We are not. We are all on the journey to find lasting peace and happiness.

Henry combines his love of metalwork artistry and therapy into his transformational metal work retreats. At present this is the only retreat of its kind in the world. As a testament to the possibilities of an empowered life, Henry runs his own FreeMind Rapid change therapy business. Henry uses hypnotherapy and talking therapy to help his clients heal past trauma and pain, which enables them to make rapid breakthroughs toward lives filled with joy and peace from the past. Henry also works for the leading holistic health care organization, spreading the message of recovery everywhere he goes.

Website: www.henryjohnstone.uk
Email: henryjohnstone.contact@gmail.com

OUT OF DARKNESS, INTO LIGHT

Tad Lusk

Depression was a strange, mysterious and devastating companion.

For a long time, I didn't even know its name. I didn't know it was a companion or a visitor--I just thought "it" was *me*.

And so, when I first started experiencing episodes of major depression as a teen, I just thought there was something wrong with *me*.

Why did I feel sad and empty for seemingly no reason? Why were there days when I couldn't bear to be around anyone, and felt inferior in every way; when just getting up and facing the day seemed like an insurmountable task?

There were indeed times when, seemingly out of nowhere, what I can only describe as a vast void would open up somewhere in my being. It was as if my mind became dark, hazy and clouded and my heart felt as heavy as a boulder and empty as a hole.

When depression visited, it would tell me horrible things about myself and about a hopeless future. It would alter my perception, drain my energy and disturb my sleep. It turned me into a different person who was irritable, cynical, and who was as unfamiliar to myself as to the people around me.

But perhaps worst of all, it infected my relationship with

myself. Depression somehow found a way to turn me against myself and convince me that I was bad, worthless, unlikeable, unlovable, defective, and so on.

Then strangely, it would disappear, occasionally just long enough for me to almost forget about the mysterious storms I had been through. For a while I would be just fine. Sometimes I would be cruising along doing great, enjoying myself, making the most of life.

But every so often, the unwanted visitor would come around and I'd be knocked right back down. Despite all my achievements, all my hard work, all the positive feedback from others, my old companion continued to haunt me.

Because I really didn't know what depression was, let alone the symptoms or causes, I never had any idea that I had "it." I just wrongly concluded that I was somehow defective. Doomed. Broken. Fucked up. It never occurred to me that I might have a diagnosable and treatable condition. So I put on a brave face and soldiered on. It hounded me through college. And after college, it became darker, heavier and more insurmountable than it had ever been.

I was living back at home, struggling to find a job, comparing myself to all my peers who were doing interesting things with their lives, and I became convinced that life had passed me by. I believed that somehow, I had failed, missed out, and that there was no hope or future for me. That's when the suicidal thoughts got worse.

I could not see a future and I could not stand the emotional pain. I wanted to feel in control of something. I wanted the people around me to know how much I was hurting because I didn't know how to communicate it or make them understand. I wanted out.

I started to daydream about how, when, and where I might end it. I thought about what I might say in a note. I thought about my funeral. But as soon as I considered the pain it would cause my family, I knew I just couldn't do it. So I would come back to reality and keep moving forward.

I remember a lot of low moments. But one in particular sticks vividly in my memory.

One night, I was crying in my bed. Our cat Sherpa came running in, leapt up on the bed and nuzzled me. He knew I was hurting and he was trying to comfort me. My dad came in to comfort me soon after, concerned and probably surprised that I was crying. All I could say through my tears was "I can't do it anymore!"

The next day I realized I was at a crossroads. Life wasn't livable in this state. I would either have to end my life by suicide or commit to somehow getting better.

So I chose the latter. I forced myself to get on the computer and search for counselors in the area. I picked up the phone and started calling, leaving messages and asking for help. I didn't realize it at the time, but that turned out to be a pivotal turning point--asking for help from a professional.

I soon started seeing a therapist nearby named Lisa, usually in the evening once a week. I barely had any money at the time, but I scraped together what I could to pay for the appointments myself. Thankfully the office worked with me to set a reasonable fee too.

Lisa was kind and understanding, and she gave me gentle suggestions for how I could start feeling better, little bit by little bit. She helped me question what I soon came to realize were the skewed thoughts and beliefs depression had convinced me of over the years. With Lisa's help, I also realized that perhaps my thoughts weren't "truth," but rather just distorted perspectives that I could change.

It soon felt like a safe haven and I started to look forward to my therapy appointments with Lisa. I always felt some relief and some hope afterward--something I hadn't felt in a long time.

Therapy also helped lead me to another huge realization: I had a condition called "Major Depressive Disorder."

I started reading articles online describing the causes and symptoms of major depression. It was everything I had experienced and struggled with to a "T." Suddenly, it all made sense. All the pieces fit.

The mercurial, unknown companion that had plagued me all those years--that I had mistakenly thought was something wrong with me--had a name. It was something *other* than me. In fact, *it wasn't me at all.* It was just something I was experiencing, something I had struggled with. But it wasn't who I was and it didn't have to define me.

I can't describe the sense of relief and validation this opened up.

On Lisa's recommendation, I also got evaluated for medication, as studies had shown that a combination of consistent therapy and an effective medication was one of the most effective ways to treat depression.

Prozac didn't work. But Pristiq--and later, Effexor--did. The lows weren't quite as low, and generally I felt a little bit lighter.

The medication wasn't a panacea, of course. I still had to work hard in therapy, and especially during my weeks in between the therapy sessions.

But it worked. Gradually my mood and outlook improved and I started to feel better more of the time. The suicidal thoughts became more faint, more fleeting, more seldom, until eventually they weren't there at all. There were still ups and downs, but after many months, I felt better able to handle them.

At some point, Lisa and I were talking and realized my mood had been positive more often than not for quite a while, so we started spacing out our sessions. Occasionally I would have a setback, but was able to rebound fairly quickly with Lisa's help and my newfound coping skills.

Eventually, Lisa and I agreed that I had reached my therapy goals. I was finally healthy in my mind, moods and functioning.

Even more importantly, I knew as certainly as I've ever known anything, that depression *wasn't me*. It was a shadowy phantom--a cunningly deceptive and powerful one--but a phantom nonetheless.

On some level, I knew I was free. I had a new life. While I knew there would still be the waves that life inevitably brings, I was pretty confident that I could handle them without drowning. And I knew that if I ever did start to struggle, I could always come back and get help.

The experience opened my eyes in so many ways. I became fascinated with mental health and started reading books on cognitive behavior therapy (CBT), self-help, meditation and spirituality.

Eventually, I was inspired to give back the gift I'd been given. So I went to graduate school to get my master's degree in Counseling Psychology and become a therapist.

It's now been over 10 years since I worked with Lisa. I've been a therapist and coach for eight years and have had the privilege of helping hundreds, if not thousands of people find solace, hope, healing and new life.

My own journey of personal growth and spiritual development continues, as it will for the rest of my life. The beautiful moments of life I'm so grateful for have been too numerous to name or count. Most have been the simple, small, everyday moments of beauty or enjoyment that make up so much of life. And some have been momentous milestones and experiences.

I've gotten to tour the country, and the world, playing guitar--performing with amazing musicians and people in some of the greatest venues, and recording numerous albums.

I've been able to spend countless holidays and birthdays with family, basking in laughter and love.

I've made lasting, meaningful friendships.

I've soaked in awe-inspiring natural beauty while hiking and traveling.

I've had a rewarding career that continues to grow and evolve.

I even got engaged to my soulmate, Jennie, on top of a mountain on the 4th of July, and will be getting married in a beautiful ceremony this summer.

Throughout it all, I've reflected on how grateful I am that I chose life over death; that I chose to step out of darkness and into light--even if I didn't know how to find it at first.

I'm so glad that I made the choice to pick up the phone and call for help. Because I never would have experienced any of these countless wonderful moments had I ended my life all those years ago.

These days, I feel a lightness, inner freedom, happiness and love for life. And while I would never wish depression on anyone, the appreciation I have for life now is in some ways deepened and made richer by knowing what it means to be lost in darkness, and by having overcome depression.

And if I can do it, you can too. Depression--and in fact, most mental health conditions are entirely treatable. Often it just starts with a choice and a phone call.

I hope that my story helps you. I hope it gives encouragement and inspiration. Most of all, I hope my story shines a light; because In the presence of light, darkness ceases to be.

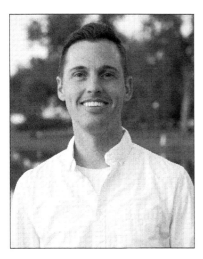

ABOUT TAD LUSK

Tad is a licensed professional counselor (LPC), personal transformation coach, musician and entrepreneur. Tad's mission is to bring healing, light, inspiration and consciousness into the world.

To learn more, visit tadlusk.com or join Tad in his free Facebook communities, Empowered Introvert Entrepreneurs and Mental Health Mastery.

www.facebook.com/groups/empoweredintrovertentrepreneurs
www.facebook.com/groups/mhmastery

"SHE WAS A DANGER TO HERSELF" TIPPED ME OVER THE EDGE

Loraine Marshall

Just over 30 years ago I had an experience that most likely changed my life.

I was just 27 years old at the time. My youngest daughter had only just entered infant's school at 4 years old. She was very small and was only just learning speech. She had difficulties because we discovered her hearing was not 100%. She had already had one operation to put in a tiny grommet and drain her eardrum after she had been diagnosed with glue ear.

At this time I had started a part-time college course to retake English at O level and I was taking driving lessons, and to top it off I had just landed a part-time job in a new bar as a kitchen assistant.

Lots going on, all moving in a positive direction. However, one day during the lunch period at the school my youngest daughter somehow managed to walk out of the schoolyard. A school assistant was calling her to return, but she didn't turn around and just kept on walking.

My husband and I were summoned to a meeting at the school where we sat in the office of the headmistress to be told what had happened and that they were unable to keep her at school meals because, as the Headmistress said, "she was a danger to herself." That short sentence stuck in my heart and mind. I could not believe she had said that. Our small daughter was in their care and was 4 years old.

Over the next few days, I tried to continue as normal, juggling college, a part-time job, driving lessons, child care, and looking after the family. I guess I may have been juggling a little too much. I could not seem to sleep for thoughts racing in my head. The headmistress' statement would not leave my thoughts. I recall making a lot of telephone calls to seek advice from a health provisional, our doctor and at one point; I phoned the Samaritan's helpline. None of this was doing me any good.

I cannot recall the timescale involved but eventually, my worried husband called out the GP. I also remember that there were other relatives in our house. I was upstairs in bed for some reason; people were coming to visit me. I could hear all the voices of people downstairs, it felt to me that all my senses were heightened. Hearing and touching definitely. I could hear what sounded like a helicopter flying overhead. I became anxious and worried. I had a feeling that I was in danger. I thought that this helicopter had been sent to spy overhead and to take me away. I remember jumping out of bed and running downstairs through the living room to the bathroom, for some reason I needed to cool down. I turned on the shower over the bath and immediately tried to climb into the bath while still clothed. This erratic behavior caused some concern. The next thing I remember was that I was in the hospital on a bed trolley with nurses and family around me.

Again lots of voices talking . . . I think I was trying to communicate to tell them that they should be asking me the questions, as the nurse was asking my husband everything.

Then I really can't recall anything more of what happened from being in the main Sunderland General hospital to waking up in a different place in the Psychiatric hospital in the district of Ryhope on the outskirts of the City.

This was how my mind and body had shut down or reacted to a situation that had caused me some stress and sleepless nights. I have no idea how long I was asleep or in a daze. What I do know is that someone would come to wake me and ask me if I wanted to eat. Sometimes I was unable even to move off the bed, so I guess I did not get food to eat regularly and was possibly just left to rest and sleep.

I can recall something of a dream or what I call a happening which seemed so real; I have talked to people in my family about this event. I believe that my spirit drifted out of my body, that I was rising upwards and then there was someone there to meet me. They told me, "No, you have to go back." This happened over and over. When I did finally get up off the bed I remember standing, looking into a long mirror on the wall. I had trousers on and a jumper. It was very strange, as the person looking back at me from the mirror looked different. The clothes I had on were very loose on my body. I took my left hand and caught the top of my trouser waistband and pulled on it. When I looked into the mirror there were at least three inches of material hanging away from my waist. I was shocked that I had lost so much weight.

I guess I was on a lot of medication at that time. The medication kept me drowsy and calm, but also confused and not able to think very clearly.

My husband and my close relatives would come to sit with me at visiting time. I don't think I was able to hold a conversation, I could hardly think straight. This one particular day I was becoming agitated because other patients had visitors and I did not. My mind started to race at the thought that I had been left there in the hospital and no one was coming to visit. I kept looking at my watch and checking the corridor, but there was no sign of my family. I decided to take matters into my own hands; I checked the doors in the corridor and found one open door so I walked out into the gardens. I knew where I was and it was a long walk home. I was prepared to start on the long journey home. I started walking away from the main building and through the grounds however, I was spotted and very soon I had three or four nurses or whoever was hurrying after me. They caught up to me and grabbed my arms as they started to walk or drag me back to the main building. It was all a bit of a drama and a commotion. I had no idea what was happening. I was pushed down over the side of the bed and all I remember was a hypodermic needle going into my buttock, then of course I was out of it again.

It took days to recover from that little episode. My feet and legs felt like lead weights, so walking was more of a shuffle. It made me feel like I was a very old woman of 80 or 90 years. To this day I have no idea what medications they were giving me or what they injected me with. I am very careful about taking prescription medication now, the main reason is that before I was married, I was poisoned by antibiotics, mainly Penicillin, and later after my first child was born Penicillin based products as well.

This was my experience of hospitalization and treatment in the UK back in 1988. How did I recover? What actions did I take? It was weeks later that I was eventually allowed to go outside into the community, but only for half a day, a sort of staged rehabilitation. I was able to go out and have lunch with relatives, my husband, and our daughters. I remember that I was given a diagnosis by the Psychiatric Hospital doctor, a term that meant nothing to me, that I could not understand. I was told that I was a "manic depressive." I was also told that I would need to take medication for the rest of my life. In my head, I was saying "no, no, no."

I was being told that I would need to take something called "Lithium salts," that the medication would require being monitored and the dosage adjusted and that I would need a regular blood test. Again in my mind, I was saying "no, no, no."

Later, on one of my allowed home visits, where I could

spend a day or two back home to see how I was coping, I got out the large volume of the medical dictionary that we had in the bookcase. I started to research the terms "manic depression" and "bipolar." The information that I was researching didn't fill me with any hope whatsoever. I didn't see myself as the person who had an illness that required medication for life.

I also did not like the idea that I may not be able to keep a driving license that I was working so hard to obtain. It may have been at this point that I made a decision, I was not going to take any more medication at the hospital. I hated how my mind seemed confused, I hated how it felt like I had cotton wool in my brain.

Back in the hospital the nurses would come out with the trolley and one by one administer the medication to all of the patients in the ward. I had made my decision and I was sticking to it. I took the tablet and put it in my mouth, I took a mouthful of water and swallowed, but the tablet was under my tongue. I would then walk away and remove the tablet and dispose of it. Rightly or wrongly I was doing things my way. I didn't feel frightened or scared. I felt that I was taking back control, enough was enough. I wanted to get out of this place.

I do not know how long it took me to start to feel better in myself, but I kept up with my decision not to take the medications that were being given to me.

What I can still recall is that one day the senior manager was on the ward. I thought to myself, I need to speak to her. I remember feeling a little anxious at that thought. I plucked up the courage and walked over to where she was. My palms were sticky with sweat. I can vaguely recall that I told her that I needed to talk. I told her that I had not been taking the medications. I told her that I felt better. I told her that this was the real me speaking. I held out my hands and said "look, my palms are clammy just at the thought of speaking to you."

It wasn't much longer after that revelation that I was

being discharged from the hospital and given some follow-up appointments. I did attend those follow-up appointments, but nothing ever came from them.

I did not need to take any medications, I did not need to have regular blood tests and take "lithium salts" for the rest of my life. I had survived an episode of being hospitalized as a medical emergency. I had survived being "sectioned" because of my attempt to "escape." However, I did have some concerns for a very long time while raising my young family. Would I ever be able to do anything in a career, hold down a job or even earn a living for myself? My self-esteem had been impacted by this episode in my life. It was my belief that I did not have any mental illness. My own GP had spoken about the episode as a "nervous breakdown," my body shutting down to protect itself.

I firmly believe that what I experienced was a normal response to some of the adversities that I had experienced in my earlier life. And because I had not slept for a number of days, my mind became disorientated. Then somehow everything just hit me all at once. So in my mind, I did not accept the diagnosis of "manic depressive" and mental illness. On the subject of medication, throughout my life I have been skeptical about medications. I am in fact allergic to Penicillin. I found this out when I was 18 years of age. I had a terrible experience of being poisoned by the prescription I had been given. I have to be really ill and suffering a lot of pain before I will seek help from the medical profession. I have not experienced any need for medical interventions since the diagnosis I was given at 27 years of age. I have managed very well without any prescription drugs.

Luckily, I managed to fully recover and rebuild my self-esteem and eventually move into a paying job, even if it was part-time and working in a supermarket. There were bigger things to come and throughout my life I have moved from one job and career to another. I have a positive outlook on life and I've studied various personal growth, mindset and self-help materials, which I believe helped me. Persistence, belief in yourself, and knowing that whatever experience or challenge you encounter is just another phase of your life and you are stronger than you think.

Through volunteering in Advice Work to becoming a Project Fundraiser in Youth & Community Charitable Organizations, plus studying with Open University and being the first of the family to earn a Bachelor of Science Honor's degree. Going on to work in higher education and then local government in the field of European Funding, to starting and running my own business in Property Management. That has all been part of my journey so far, and now another change, another new episode. I am writing a book of my story "What Type Of Man," the story of betrayal, infidelity, discard and abandonment.

ABOUT LORAINE MARSHALL

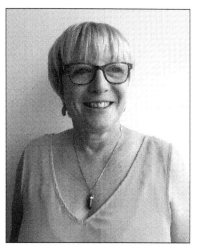

Currently, I do not have a job, I do not have an income-generating business yet. I'm living in the countryside of Cartagena in the property that my now ex-partner Paul purchased in 2015. I am on a mission of discovery, after being abruptly discarded by my ex in August 2020.

I was a property manager working my own business in Letting and Property Management. I had built up that business from scratch. I started the business in 2005 when I was with my previous partner John, before he died of a heart attack at the young age of 52 years. I let that business go in 2016 when I moved to Spain, selling the clients' database and rent book to another agent in my hometown of Sunderland.

While living in Spain I have enjoyed Yoga classes, Spanish lessons, art classes, and even took part in the Cartagena Dance Carnival in February 2020, I was involved in dance practices for four months leading up to the carnival parade. It was the first time that I had done anything like this before, at 59 years of age dancing through the city streets for two and a half hours. I loved it. I also love to get out into the grounds of the villa and work on transforming the land, laying paths, planting trees, creating planted areas with yuccas, aloes, cactus and other Spanish garden shrubs, which I don't think of as work. Career wise I am writing my first book and working on following my passion to create multiple streams of online income.

WHAT A PICKLE!

Diane Mintz

Why did it take a trip to a psychiatric hospital for me to hear that I had a substance abuse problem? I finally agreed to commit myself after two months of battling debilitating depression. I could not function and believed I never would again. I could not see a flicker of light at the end of the dark tunnel.

Drugs and alcohol had been my go-to remedy for everything since I was sixteen, but it sure seemed as though I was having a great time when I was partying with friends. A chaotic relationship and painful broken marriage engagement sent me down that dark spiral. It was the second time we had called off the wedding. Well, the third time if you count when the church burnt down.

Suicidal thoughts weighed heavily on my tortured mind before entering the hospital and only got worse because I believed that I would forever have "mental patient" branded on my forehead. A mental patient with a serious secondary problem without a solution. You see, they didn't provide treatment for addiction in the psych ward back then. They left me to figure that one out on my own.

My solution was to end my life. I stole my dad's pain pills and checked myself into a hotel room where I was going to permanently check out. If the pills chased down with a bottle of liquor didn't kill me, they would get me numb enough to carry out my main plan—to slash my wrist. It was a genuine miracle that I survived.

Seeing the fear and pain in my family's eyes shook me up. I never wanted to do that again, but it was no surprise that I returned to the temporary fix of drugs and alcohol to stifle my pain. This time I had other chemicals on board. The antidepressants together with my substance potpourri sent me soaring into my first manic episode.

The manic feeling was familiar to me because I enjoyed drugs that gave me a similar high, but the euphoric sensation didn't wear off. It was astonishing to come out such a dense, mind-numbing fog into such remarkable clarity. This time, after many sleepless nights, it turned into psychosis. Thus, my next trip to the psych ward.

My bipolar roller coaster ride went on for ten relentless years. I enjoyed the thrills, but it never ended well. Depression always followed my manic runs fueled by the humiliation from my delusional and grandiose behavior.

One problem was that I didn't think I was a "real" alcoholic because I was able to control my drinking when my moods weren't running amok. Fortunately, the only requirement for Alcoholics Anonymous was a *desire* to stop drinking. So, I attended meetings. Unfortunately, I encountered some twelve-steppers who convinced me not to take my mood stabilizing psychotropic medications. They believed, "A drug is a drug."

I was in and out of AA, skipping steps, missing steps, side-stepping, and half-stepping on a rapidly revolving dance floor that spun me round and round. I was alternately drinking, using, depressed, or manic. I inevitably wound up back where I started. Dual diagnosis treatment was what I needed, but it was unheard of at the time. Recovery seemed impossible when it was left up to me, the impaired one, to integrate my ping pong treatment from AA to psych doctors. I was either too depressed to follow the directions of the twelve-step program or was too manic to care. Either way, my mind got in the way of treatment.

You may be surprised to know that I was only unemployed a short time prior to my first hospitalization and had a great job during thirteen of the years that I struggled the most. Spotting mental illness and addiction is not as obvious as it seems. I surrounded myself with other drinkers and blended in like a chameleon. I didn't realize that alcoholism was rampant in my extended family. I didn't know the signs and the consequences were always hidden. Everyone around me made drinking look social and fun. I didn't see much of the downside.

It was so difficult on my family when I didn't see the need for treatment, but they never gave up on me. My ups and downs of partying often masked and mimicked my psychiatric symptoms. I enjoyed alcohol and the drugs I chose because I thought they made me more social and interesting. It was counterintuitive to take prescriptions that didn't give me that desired feeling.

What made matters worse was a symptom of my mania that we didn't know about at the time. It is an unawareness syndrome called anosognosia. When I was manic, aside from enjoying the euphoric feeling, my brain literally couldn't recognize a problem. Anosognosia was cruel and unusual punishment for anyone trying to convince me that I needed treatment, especially because my judgment was so impaired that I ended up in some very dangerous, almost fatal, situations.

I wish I had realized that I needed to be sober, whether I was an alcoholic or not, because my random drug use and drinking was dangerous with my brain chemistry. I simply could not balance my moods when I drank and used drugs. A twelve-step friend helped me by suggesting that I consider myself allergic to alcohol and recreational drugs. That helped me stay away from friends who didn't understand or respect my allergy. Everyone knows to be careful around someone with peanut allergies because bad things happen to them. It was the same with me and alcohol.

I wish it had been impressed upon me that all recreational drugs and alcohol were off-limits for me simply because I have a serious mood disorder. I couldn't just add random doses of mood-altering substances and expect to stay in balance. Instead, some mental health professionals told me that I "could drink in moderation." Moderation? Moderation meant very different things to me when I felt so different all the time. Why would they trust me to be able to manage that? I didn't trust myself.

After many failed attempts, I got sober in AA in 1991. I have taken my mood stabilizing medication faithfully and have stayed within a manageable mood zone ever since. I am not cured. To think along those lines would tempt me to drink or go off my meds. No more hospitals or life-disrupting chaos.

When my compulsion to drink finally lifted and the monkey on my back stopped breathing down my neck, I felt liberated. But new challenges were just around the corner. After I was two years sane and sober, I fell in love with a man in a twelve-step program who had a similar past as mine. He was very committed to recovery, but his diagnosis was a complete mystery until after we were married. However, that's another story. One so unique I was compelled to write, *In Sickness and in Mental Health: Living with and Loving Someone with Mental Illness*.

Greg's illness has been quite a challenge over the twenty-plus years we have been together, but the fact that I had experience in recovery from mental illness gave me a unique sensitivity. I understood that my husband's struggles and problems were due to a mental illness so I could help him get treatment. I have advocated for mentors and peers for everyone. It is hard enough to jump though the mental health maze to get treatment when one feels well. Frankly, it is too difficult for someone to even recognize what the problem is by themselves. We can't recognize brain issues with a brain that is having issues!

People are shocked when they learn that I live a stable life with bipolar disorder, and my husband has lived with schizoaffective disorder for over thirty years. It is amazing to think of how debilitated by mental illness and addiction we once were. We should have been homeless, institutionalized, or dead. Yet we are two ordinary people living extraordinary lives. We have two great kids and started our own IT Company in 2005.

I enjoy my work in mental health the most. I run focus groups for Medi-Cal mental health and substance abuse clients and volunteer and sit on the board for The National Alliance on Mental Illness NAMI Sacramento. The biggest blessing was when I began speaking on three speakers' bureaus in 2014. Many years ago, when my husband and I began to disclose to friends and talk about our conditions, we were shocked to receive acceptance and compassion. They may not have understood, but their acceptance did wonders for our mental health. It accelerated our recovery!

I speak candidly and unashamedly to whoever will listen about the very thing I kept secret for so long. I believed that I needed to hide my condition, or I would feel worse about myself because of the stigma I feared. My big secret was a major hindrance that prolonged my ability to recover. What a welcome surprise to receive positive feedback and encouragement from everyone. People would come to find out that we are people with misunderstood, incurable conditions living in long-term recovery. Our story has helped people who used to be hiding and limping through life.

Other speakers agree that sharing their experience has been a major factor in their personal healing and recovery. We also encourage and support each other so that we can grow and heal in ways we didn't think possible. When we share with someone, even on a one-to-one basis, it may seem like a drop in a big ocean of stigma and misinformation, but for every person we reach there is a ripple effect. This is the outside impact. The surprising changes happen on the inside when we experience the freedom of breaking free of shame and experience the power of making a difference in the lives of others.

If my dream came true, people who are addicted or mentally ill would never be thought of as "losers" or "worthless" but as amazing brave warriors who have ruthless invisible foes to conquer. Sadly, I am not alone to have felt the hopelessness and condemnation from without and within. We wonder, "Am I just weak-willed?" It was so frustrating to think I just needed to try harder. It made my condition worse. If society still imposes on us that getting psychiatric help is weak, naturally people will continue to self-medicate. If two powerful forces like that feed on each other it can be double trouble.

Our wellness is all about balance. Greg and I both require medicine and therapy along with spiritual development, connection, and growth to remain sober and sane. We are always grateful for our sobriety. Some people can't fathom the notion of living without alcohol. They ask, "Surely you can have a little celebratory champagne at a wedding, right?" Nope. For me, "One is too many and a thousand is never enough." It is the way my brain is wired. They make it very clear in AA that once we become a pickle, we can never go back to being a cucumber. I'm not embarrassed to be a pickle.

I will continue to speak publicly about our experience to bring about a change of perception, so we can eradicate negative judgment towards people with mental illness and addiction. Judge bad behavior, not the person. Apply consequences, not condemnation. Treat those who struggle with these mind-boggling problems with compassion and respect. When we get support and acceptance from the outside, our inside responds better and that's when recovery happens.

I am committed to saying proudly that there is no shame in having my conditions. Mine is not a dreary life sentence. There is hope. Recovery does happen. With the right treatment and support, even pickles with mental illness like me can live full abundant lives.

In Sickness and in Mental Health is available on Amazon, Barnes and Noble, and Smashwords.

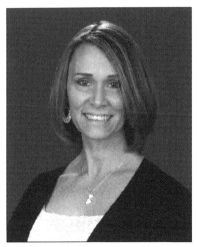

ABOUT DIANE MINTZ

Diane is the author of the book, *In Sickness and in Mental Health—Living with and Loving Someone with Mental Illness* and owner of Mintz Computer Guyz along with her husband Greg.

She serves on the board for the Sacramento National Alliance on Mental Illness and is a Consumer Family Member Consultant for a behavioral health external quality review organization.

Diane has been a pioneer in sharing publicly about her bipolar disorder. She has done over one hundred presentations to a wide variety of audiences since 2014. Her mission is to give a new perspective of mental illness and addiction; one that inspires society to support the afflicted and give everyone hope for recovery.

More at www.dianemintzauthor.com

100% sales donated to NAMISacramento

CHAOS TO COURAGE, A JOURNEY OF HOPE!

Mehreen Siddiqui

I still remember every detail as if it were today. In my mind's eye, I see the bright pink flowers on my mother's blouse and hear her high heels clicking as she strode confidently towards my dad's house. Her sweet floral perfume wafted into the cool autumn air as deep sepia curls bounced around her beautiful, doe-like face. Bright Christian Dior lipstick and light, airy cropped pants spoke of confidence and poise.

Behind her, I followed hesitantly, fearfully. After leaving us a few years ago, my dad had gone back to his homeland of Pakistan, found a new wife, and brought her to the states. Today, my mother had decked herself in her best clothes to take us to see our new stepmom.

"How are you?" My mother addressed her rival as we entered the house. "I just wanted to come here today and meet you."

I sat stiffly on the couch, baffled by the strangeness of it all. Why were my mother and dad calmly conversing in the same room? Before the divorce, shouting and screaming were the only sounds we heard when they were together.

I smiled nervously, looking from person to person. Why had

my mother decided to bring us here? After an awkward period of tense formalities, my mother left.

It was late at night when my dad dropped us off at home. The stilted, uncomfortable visit with my stepmom was over, and I was ready to be home. The haunting call of a night bird hung in the cool Arkansas evening as I opened the door to my home.

As soon as I stepped into the foyer, I knew something was wrong. An ominous heaviness surrounded me like the cold, clammy night air. Glancing toward the stairs that wound upwards to the right, I glimpsed the cause of my foreboding. My mother sprawled on the stairs, head down. Her legs were lifelessly draped on the upper stairs. With her face staring up at the ceiling, legs exposed, and maxi-dress nightgown billowing around her, she presented the picture of despair.

My mother was wailing. My grandfather stood over her, splashing water on her face.

"See, look at your mother," he accused. "Who's going to take care of her now? Your father went and remarried, and just look at your mother now. She's completely out of it."

Looking on helplessly, unsure how to make the situation better, I vowed that I would never, ever become as dependent on another person as my mother had been on my dad. I would never allow a loss or a separation to tear me apart like that.

My mind went into high gear.

"How can I fix this?" I wondered. It was a question I would continue to ask many times in the upcoming months.

For years, I experienced the roller coaster of my mother's manic and depressive states. Her struggle with bipolar schizoaffective disorder had begun with postpartum depression shortly after my birth, but it had worsened when she and my father divorced. The roller coaster felt less like an amusement park ride and more like a derailed train hurtling towards destruction.

Living with an angry, irrational, and manic mother was stressful. I never knew how she would react or what mood she would be in. She tried hard to be a good mother, frequently apologizing for the ways she failed to take care of us. Mother often acted like a small child, leaning on us for comfort. Other times, she said unspeakable things to us girls, treating us harshly. Despite the constant turmoil, I told myself this was normal.

Throughout my childhood, no one told us the truth about our mother. When she spent three months in the psychiatric ward, we were told she went to see her sister in India. Our uncle and grandparents finally allowed us to visit her in the hospital, but they warned us not to tell anyone where she was. They lied saying that, if we did tell, our dad would get custody of us and we would be sent back to Pakistan. Without help or accurate information, my sisters and I did the best we could to cope on our own.

For me, coping meant becoming invisible and doing my best. If I got good grades, I could avoid triggering my mother's erratic meltdowns. Throughout my childhood, I kept my home life and school life separate. I had many surface-level friendships that distracted me from the yelling and beatings that went on at home. But I never invited my friends to visit, and none of them knew what went on behind closed doors.

When my mother was in her manic state, she would go on spending sprees. Hours later, she would come home loaded down with name-brand makeup, fancy clothes, sparkling jewelry, and any household items that had struck her fancy. When she arrived home, my dad would become irate. He was a surgeon and well to do, but he didn't approve of such irrational spending. Often, the fights would turn violent.

I remember an epic tussle that started on the way out of Service Merchandise. The red arches and the white pillars of the store are seared into my memory as I focused to block out the yelling and screaming. The fight continued all the way out to the parking lot and into the car. It was the last fight they had. My father realized he couldn't control her spending. Quickly, he escaped the marriage with his checkbook and his sanity.

Later, I blamed my dad and my stepmother for my mother's downward spiral. I reasoned that my mother fell apart because dad left and moved on with his life. My 12-year-old brain couldn't distinguish between reality and fiction when my grandfather blamed the entire situation on my dad and his new wife.

It wasn't until college that I realized the true cause of my mother's suffering. In a psychology class, I read about schizophrenia and bipolar. Stunned, I said to myself, "This is my mother." Immediately calling my uncle, I explained what I'd learned.

"Yeah, we know," he replied dispassionately. "How was I supposed to explain that to a twelve-year-old?"

As I became a young adult, my coping strategy was to block my memories. Until my mother died at age 55, many of these memories were safely locked away in a place that no one could access, not even myself. I constantly focused on the future and on taking care of myself and everyone around me. I was a bossy overachiever who strove for perfection in everything.

Some of my memories of my mother were sweet and lovely. She was a talented artist and painter. Mother loved red roses and monarch butterflies. Intelligent and beautiful, she was on the Dean's list in school. When my mother met my husband's parents for the first time, she invited us to a lavish spread of food. Serving dinner on her finest china, she pulled out all the stops to make us feel welcome. When I had children of my own, she held them lovingly and took care of me after my children's birth. There were a few moments that felt normal, even beautiful.

But when she died, my world came crashing down. A different Mehreen woke up the day after mother passed. Floods of emotion and memory washed over me with hurricane force. As I began reliving her life in my head, the horrific memories started resurfacing. *How could she have beat us like that? How could she have said those things to us? That's messed up! I have children. I would never treat my children this way. What the heck?*

One night, my husband found me staring at the wall, trembling.

"They beat us, they hurt us," I was saying over and over in shock.

When I realized the toll my past was taking on my life and marriage, I threw my energy into getting help. For four years, I worked on healing myself and my story. It was hard to find a therapist who understood the dynamics of my Pakistan-American background, but I finally found one. She helped me talk about the past trauma so I could heal from it. My counselor gave me a safe space to talk about what happened.

During that time, I also went to a marriage counselor. I wanted to save my precarious, insecure marriage. Realizing that my past was jeopardizing my relationship with the man I loved best, I worked hard to fix my marriage. But I wasn't sure how.

In 2018, I discovered a powerful course that changed the way I viewed my entire life: Landmark Forum. As if a switch were flipped, a light came on in my brain. Landmark Forum's catchphrase is, "Redefine the very nature of what's possible." It certainly reframed life for me; it was the best thing I ever did.

As I soaked in the transformational teaching of the Landmark Forum session, something dawned on me. *I can choose who I am.* In the past, I had re-enacted learned behaviors that I absorbed from my mother. She had taught me seemingly immutable lessons:

People leave you.

You can't trust men.

People will only betray you and take your money.

These lessons were not only unhelpful, but they were also not true of my present life. My mother may have experienced rejection and betrayal, but I was experiencing a safe, loving husband. The messages I listened to every day had nothing to do with my current life, and they had everything to do with my mother's past life.

As I realized that my paranoia was not who I really was, I began to be present to the source of my thoughts. I started to change where my thoughts originated from. My marriage transformed, my relationships changed, and I began to see myself in a new light.

I'm still doing the never-ending work of healing, but I've come a long way. I'm much more aware of who I am, and I want to do whatever it takes to change the family tree. I am healing from generational trauma so I don't pass it on to my children and grandchildren.

In 2017, my sisters and I started a nonprofit organization to help others who had the same story as we did. We named our nonprofit after our mother, SEEMA. The acronym stands for Support Embrace Empower Mental Health Advocacy. We help people understand and eradicate the stigma of mental health. We also encourage caregivers of people struggling with mental health.

In addition, I coach high achieving, successful women who are experiencing burn out. My business, Goal Set Coach, helps women who are running on fumes. What started as a passion for these women has devolved into an exhausting source of burn out, and I help them get their joy back.

I can see myself in these women. Many of them are consumed with pleasing people and perfectionism because of their own traumatic past. Together, we work to set them free and help them find their identity.

I explain to these women what I have learned over a lifetime: I must keep showing up for others. I need to trust others and allow people to contribute to me. I'm speaking to myself as well as to these beautiful women: we all must take care of ourselves first. Just because we're not doing something doesn't mean we're not being productive. Sometimes, wonderful things happen in their own time without us doing anything at all. We can trust that being ourselves is beautiful. We are lovable, just as we are.

ABOUT MEHREEN SIDDIQUI

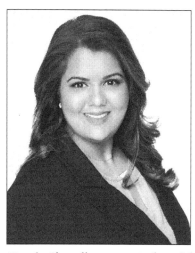

Mehreen has been married to her college sweetheart for twenty years. She has two daughters, ages 15 and 18. She has been a consultant for 16 years in corporate America. More recently, she started a nonprofit that advocates for mental health. She is also the CEO of a thriving coaching business for overwhelmed high-achieving women, Goal Set Coach. She tells women it doesn't have to be "stressful to be successful." They can achieve balance, health, and wholeness in every area of their lives. Learn more by visiting ileadwithexcellence.com.

THE SOUL'S JOURNEY: FROM DARKNESS TO LIGHT

Susan Sims Hillbrand

U nderstanding and intertwining the complexity of what happened through two stories and another yet to be known. My story today differs from the original diagnosis. Accepting what the allopathic doctors told me, taking the medications, receiving individual and group therapy, and believing I was branded for life, I knew deep down there was more to uncover and discover. I am not saying they got it wrong. I am here to say there is more to know. I spent 24 years carrying the original story that served me well. It was a journey of discomfort that led me through an amazing exploration as I questioned what happened to me. In the emergency room of a hospital my husband is told I am having a manic episode known then as Manic Depressive Illness, now known as Bi-Polar Disorder. It went from being called an illness to a disease or is it both? The allopathic medical community was and still is trying to grasp the complexity of this societal taboo called Mental Illness or is it Mental Health? BTW the name needs an upgrade, there is too much baggage attached. Do we have a health care system or a sick care system? Our system is failing to be a whole body, mind and spirit course of action.

Yes, I was functioning, not having any more severe episodes and yet still holding a heavy discomfort. Something was pushing me to change the story by understanding it from a deeper level, another perspective or perhaps seeing it from another dimension. I was thrown over the threshold that day in 1991. My identity was shattered. I didn't know who or what to trust. I feared I had died and gone to hell. This is called, Dark Night of the Soul, a spiritual crisis, and I call it Spiritual Emergence.

Let's go back to the original story as there are more years of misunderstanding and unhealthy thinking than the number of years since I healed the wound by choosing another way of seeing it. Although time doesn't matter, where I am today and how I got to this healthy state of being does. I remember the discomfort as a child and having a strong sense I had an inner knowing, a deeper intelligence, higher self, the divine within trying to speak to me. Of course I did not have those words to express the feeling, just a deep knowing that something was there. It felt distant and not accessible. Like there was an empty space in my gut. Nobody talked about the divine realm within. As a child so many things, people and situations form and inform us, but not how to honor and trust your inner knowing. I felt different, misunderstood, not school smart, unheard and very alone, yet I was outgoing and good at sports. No one knew how lost and alone I felt. I was good at disguising my inner turmoil then soothing it later as a teenager using drugs and alcohol. They call that self-medicating. Moving forward twenty years later from my teen years, married with two beautiful children, I was being placed in the psychiatric ward of a hospital given a label with instructions to take and do what the doctors say in order to cope and return to my family. We were all in shock and thanks to a good friend's recommendation the kids and my husband went for therapy, but there was still a lot to adjust to and understand. I was happy to know why I had been self-medicating thinking I finally had an answer. It didn't take long for the branding of mental illness to sink in. Feeling trapped in a container, losing friends, and becoming paranoid that everyone could see I was not right perhaps even crazy. There were friends who cared and supported me. The label was a mixed blessing and one that needed exploring. My parents didn't want to accept my condition. Mental illness . . . not our daughter. They hoped a few therapy sessions would cure me. A year later my mother told me to stop therapy because it can be addictive. Therapy was extremely helpful yet even the therapists could only take me so far. The last therapist suggested I was afraid to do my art because, here comes another stigma, I thought being an artist meant I must be crazy. At the time I was not able to produce new work.

Over the river and through the woods, into the cave and out again I travelled. I weaned off medication with professional guidance and continued therapy until I was ready to take a new path. I had a team of support who recognized I was ready to start anew. I worked hard to get to that healing place with many ups and downs, yet I was still holding the wounded story. It would take another 10 years to find the new one and release the older version that no longer served me. During a workshop with the marvelous Jean Houston, a legend in her own time as a world renowned scholar, futurist, and researcher in human capacities, social change, and systemic transformation, the new story emerged. As an Evolutionary Pioneer I was drawn to explore the weekend workshop not knowing I was about to rewrite my history/her-story. We were to take an unpleasant experience and change the way we were telling the story through play acting imagination. I chose to create a new story from research about older cultures and the revered Shamans. Instead of doctors coming to my rescue it was a shaman and team of wisdom keepers who took me to the forest, not a hospital, to sit by a fire blindfolded so as to not lose sight of the inner experience as I was being initiated, not medicated, into the full potential of spirit. They were an indigenous wisdom tribe who knew the ancient signs well of one who is touched by the spirit. I received tender loving support and guidance on how to enter the Dark Night of the Soul in a safe place for my initiation and soul journey. Seeing my experience as a Spiritual Emergence no longer trapped in an old paradigm of outdated thinking I felt lighter, free and open to embody who I/we truly are—spiritual beings having a spiritual experience in human form. The human part is complex and lives within many contextual experiences. Our relationship to mental illness is connected to our unhealthy culture.

Childhood experiences good and not so good, positive and negative, and our natural instincts get repressed and are stored in our subconscious. Our true nature gets stuck in the shadowy realms of misunderstandings. Those of us who are touched are sensitive and easily triggered by others' energies that become infused with our energy field. What have we been exposed to in life? How do we set up our boundaries of protection? It becomes a challenge to heal when we are given mixed messages, too much, too little or the wrong medication and therapy that no longer serves the needs of today's complexities. We are evolving into a new self and we must recognize the next story to support the transition. Once we gain a healthy relationship with our higher self the suffering transforms into a person who can be a spiritual anchor for the world. Now more than ever our world needs us. Are we provided with the tools to transform? The mystery to why some can heal and others suffer a lifetime continues to be explored yet we as a society need to see the highest possible good, provide tender loving care, be understanding, listen and be inquisitive, not afraid of those who are considered mentally ill. There is a story in each and every one of us waiting to unfold. Their condition, my condition is our/your condition. We all contribute to the insaneness and craziness of society when we turn away from and not lean into the stories of what happened. Our priorities are off base, we have lost our true nature.

I am an artist and the creative process can be very revealing.

Spending time looking at the images I had created of light beings, called *Penlight Performances*, I started to notice the art expressing the story about Spiritual Emergence. The art was ahead of me and I was now catching up to what was being expressed. Working in the dark and expressing the human form with light. Darkness to Light, oh there seems to be a theme here.

As an Artist of Possibility, a beaming enthusiastic Light Being, an Inspirational Influencer I embrace the creative Life Force Energy of the Universe and Beyond. I give talks and guide groups using my artistic expression of words and images to help unleash the creative genius that lives within us all. The journey from Darkness to Light, from Mental Illness to Spiritual Emergence is providing the opportunity to connect deeper with Life, to see and experience our interconnectedness with each other and nature. The suffering and brokenness can be patched and repaired and turned into another form of beauty. Like Wabi Sabi, the beauty of things imperfect, impermanent and incomplete. We are a paradox of perfection and imperfection, permanent and impermanent, complete and incomplete. Our eternal nature is stable and our transient being is complex and wobbly and is always in a process of entering new territory. Embrace the unknown of Life with Love and Trust. Take a deep breath, relax and explore the inner depths of who you/we truly are. Those of us who have taken the journey of healing and renewal have a responsibility to share and support one another along the path to awakened relationships with self, others and Mother Earth. Change your perspective, create your inner sanctuary, seek support, we cannot do this alone and feel your true sacred essence into your creative genius. We are on this planet together co-creating a new self within a new world where the term mental illness will be transported and transformed into mental clarity and a whole body wellness where we can thrive in a peaceful place. Imagine that world story and what is possible. We are all artists of possibility, creative expressions, storied beings, with interpenetrating souls, ready to live in our full potential. The next story to be known is unfolding.

In the Womb

As I emerge from the protective shell
the cocoon of the womb
into a world of **unrest**
I am able to be still
a healing center
in the **silence**
in the **breath**
I have arrived

ABOUT SUSAN SIMS HILLBRAND

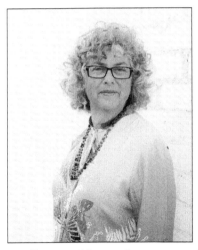

Susan is an artist creating images and poetry titling her life's work **Spiritual Matrices,** breath of the womb. She guides groups using the images and poetry to explore a co-creative conversation and how we can participate more fully as our true nature. Hillbrand expresses a spiritual landscape of a personal journey from darkness to the light. Influenced by her small town Ohio upbringing and living in urban centers on both coasts, currently LA, Hillbrand connects the symbolic relationship of our external and internal life by seeing similarities in our life experiences and our inner spiritual landscape. Her subject matter is spirit and our relationship to the evolving global community. As an art student at California State University, Northridge, where she received a BFA, Hillbrand started to explore the question, "Who are we and what are we becoming?" By outlining her body with light she saw the possibilities of illuminating the hidden spirit, and this personal exploration began as **Penlight Performances.** Her work is published in lightpaintingphotography.com, French, Italian and German art / science books and The Artist of Possibility magazine. She participates in the Mystery School membership circle bringing a new paradigm to life.

Susan Sims Hillbrand
susansimshillbrand.com

A BATTLE IN MY MIND

Christine Whitehead Lavulo

My first thoughts of suicide came when I was 13 years old. My family had just moved from the "big city" to a suburb about 20 miles north. It was like a complete culture shock. I didn't fit in and nothing felt right. I began to believe that there was a conspiracy against me even—that people were just pretending to be my friend to set me up for pain and humiliation. My mom had to go back to work full-time so she wasn't around nearly as much. Our family was having some financial challenges. I felt lonely and invisible. I figured my feelings of depression were a result of this event. Imagine my surprise when we moved back "home" to the city a few years later and the depression didn't ease up. But again, it was probably just the angst of teenage years.

I got pregnant at 17 and graduated high school with a new baby. That winter my parents decided I needed to be independent and "helped" me out the door. I was a young, single mom living completely on my own. The depression kicked in and began to feel unbearable. Thoughts of suicide would be countered by the thought of leaving my son without a mother. And even though, at times, that seemed like it would be better for him, knowing the psychological effects it could have kept me in the game.

This cycle would continue and I would continue to believe

it was "circumstantial". I just needed to find a husband, have a better job, live in a better house and so forth.

I was caught off guard when the depression hit me again at age 26. I was married, we had a house and I had two wonderful and precious sons. I had a nice job that was part time and I really enjoyed it. So how come I was finding myself crying the entire drive home from work? It didn't make sense. My life was good. I had nothing to be "sad" about. This was the point when I finally decided it was time to ask for help. I made an appointment with a primary care physician and was prescribed Prozac. And it helped . . . for a while. But at some point I began to feel . . . nothing. It was nice to not feel sad and gloomy, but I hated that I didn't feel happy either. I didn't get excited about anything. I was just numb. So I stopped taking it and I seemed to be a lot better.

When my third son was about a year old the depression hit like never before. We were living in a great apartment outside Denver, Colorado. My husband had a great job, I was able to stay home and care for my sons and we were close to my sister. Life was seemingly really good. So it was alarming to me when these feelings of depression crept back in. But they took root in a way I had never experienced before. I remember the day well. It was just me and the baby at home. For some reason motherhood just seemed hard that day. I was having a hard time being a mom at all. Everything just seemed completely overwhelming.

I felt this illogical anger and resentment towards my precious son. That led me to feeling bad about myself as a mother. Which led to me feeling unworthy to be a mother. Which spiraled down the rabbit hole of me just not being enough, not being worthy, not being important, not having a purpose and so forth. The feelings enveloped me and took hold of me. I sat there crying as I fought the thoughts of suicide, which had become a normal part of this downward spiral. "I don't want to live like this, no one would even notice if I was gone. I am going to be doing everyone a favor. My life is worthless." Those were just a few of the thoughts attacking me as I cried non-stop. And, like always, I sat and tried to dispute the negative words and reason with myself. Only this time instead of my son being a reason for me to fight to live, the thought came to my mind . . . "I can't leave my kids with the wreckage of a mom who took her own life. The only solution is to kill my kids and then myself".

Fortunately, I had just enough fortitude and strength to talk myself out of the insanity. But the thought in and of itself scared me. It rocked me to the core of my soul. I never could understand these women, like Susan Smith, who killed their children before themselves. I would think . . . "How could anyone do that to their children?" And suddenly, I understood. Several years later, a former colleague of mine actually did this. She shot her two beautiful girls and then herself. All I could think to myself is I wish I would've known she was struggling. She was always super upbeat and positive. What could I have done differently? How could I have reached her? How can I try to keep this from happening to someone else? Maybe, just maybe, if I was more open to sharing my own story, I could help give hope to those that are thinking of ending theirs.

It's hard to explain it to someone, but it seems there is a battle raging inside my mind-almost all the time. The thoughts come rapidly and it's hard for me to even grasp what I'm thinking. It becomes exhausting getting one negative thought and continually trying to counter it with the truth. "I'll never be good enough" gets changed to "I'm good enough because I'm a daughter of God. I claim the gift of grace through Christ Jesus". "No one likes me" gets changed to "It is obvious people do like you since you have friends and people seek you out". But I can't always catch all the negative thoughts to correct them. It's constant and unrelenting when it happens. It somewhat forces me to just "check out". I will find a mindless show to watch. I can't seem to do anything but lay there and try to occupy my mind with other things so I don't have to think at all, so I won't produce a negative feeling. Because those feelings can compound and become unbearable.

Every day I would begin that battle as my mind waged war against me. Some days I would wake up fine and other days I would even make it through most of the day. But then others, the thoughts would begin to assault me early in the day, which then brought out feelings I wasn't prepared to address. And most of the time, I wasn't even sure why I was feeling this way. There were many times where there was no evidence of the thoughts I was telling myself. And some days I would have these feelings with no thoughts at all. Just a sinking feeling in my chest of doom and gloom. It didn't make sense and trying to explain it to someone else seemed near impossible.

I began to really think I might be "crazy". You know, looney bin, mental hospital kind of crazy. Sometimes I would just snap—lash out, be reduced to tears, and I was doing it all to myself with no understanding and no explanation to be found.

My family is filled with "mental illness" and it's been sad to see how some people respond to it simply because they don't understand it and choose not to learn. We have to learn compassion as a society if we will ever truly put an end to the stigmas that are out there. Having challenges does not make a person unstable. It certainly doesn't make a person unlovable, but that is what most people believe about themselves because of how these challenges have been treated by people they thought loved them. Really, it was just a lack of understanding and a fear of what has been perpetuated by the media and society.

Most people who struggle with mental illness self-medicate if they do not seek professional help. Drugs, alcohol, food, sex . . . it appears easier to try and push down these feelings rather than to experience them and thus addiction starts. My son started using drugs at the age of 14. When he was 17 we took him to a psychiatrist to see about getting him diagnosed and medicated with something that could help the symptoms and allow him to better cope.

The medication they gave him was difficult for him, and I completely understood. He never felt like himself, no matter which combination they used. He would feel too sleepy, too jumpy, and in general, out of body. I had experienced that before with a medication prescribed for my anxiety and so I completely understood why he absolutely did not want to take them.

He would have these "episodes" (that's what I called them) when he would drink too much hard alcohol, which was quite possibly mixed with any other combination of illicit narcotics. He would almost seem possessed, and in many ways, I believe that's exactly what it was. When he would look at me, it was like he wasn't there. And the rage that ensued would be completely unwarranted and illogical. But he would express deep seeded emotions that just had to be let loose, even if it meant he would self-destruct. So many feelings of being unworthy, of not being enough, of feeling invisible, unheard, not validated. I completely understood. While my experiences manifested differently, I knew exactly how he felt inside.

He went to a therapist for a little while, and he did learn a few tools and techniques, but when she took another job and referred him to someone else, he didn't want to start over with building a relationship and just gave up and went back to the thing that was easiest.

We spent years on a roller coaster ride with his moods and the waves of mania and depression. But as time went on, and he got older and learned valuable and painful lessons, he became more open to what was working for me.

What was working for me, you ask? First and foremost, I would say my belief in something or someone higher than me. A higher power, God.

A lot of people want to buck religion these days and it seems like it's taboo to even talk about God, and yet our very country was founded on the basis of religious freedoms and to become "one nation under God". And so I will take this opportunity to say that without God, I believe I would be dead. It's because of His love and mercy that I have had the strength to carry on. The scriptures teach us that "with God, nothing is impossible". And I firmly believe that.

In addition to my religious convictions and relationship with God, I had a friend refer me to a massage therapist in 2004 that specialized in craniosacral therapy. If you've never experienced this, I highly recommend it. It is an energy modality, and it is used to clear energetic blocks. I had many powerful sessions in her office where so many buried things came to light and could be healed, without me having to talk about and relive it. Healing happened in so many ways.

I also started practicing more holistic habits: eating more nutritionally healthy and balanced meals, taking high-quality supplements, using essential oils and CBD oil. I started reading personal development books and learning more about myself and about habits I could incorporate into my life that could help me better cope and manage these symptoms when they came on. It made a world of difference in how I felt and how I functioned!

I want to explain something, however. You are never "cured" of mental illness. You learn how to adapt, how to cope and how to manage it.

As a matter of fact, even with how far I've come and all that I know, the past few nights were rough. The thoughts of wanting to get out of this world and away from this life were once again present. The thoughts cause me to freeze. I want to reach out to someone, find someone to talk to, just get things off my chest. But I can't seem to dial the phone. My mind will give me 3-4 people to call and I will find a "reason" why I can't call each of them. Sometimes I have reached out to someone and not gotten a response, and I think that has almost conditioned me to stop trying. It's a ridiculous thing, I know. And yet, I continue to respond in that same way. It's a weird thing too. It doesn't make sense, and I know it doesn't make sense, and yet I can't seem to change it.

Sometimes the only way to get through these days is just to allow them to happen. I allow myself to feel what I'm feeling, to think what I'm thinking, to experience everything I need to experience. I do my best to keep it from getting out of control. I use my essential oils, do my positive self-talk to the best of my abilities, I read my scriptures and say my prayers. And then I remind myself that I've been through this before, I've been through worse, and I have always gotten through it.

As they say, "this too shall pass". Knowing that the sun will rise again each morning gives me the fortitude to see the nights through. Each day gives me a new opportunity to rise up again, just as the sun does.

ABOUT CHRISTINE LAVULO

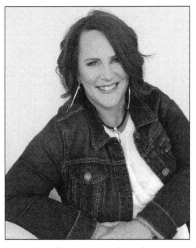

Christine is a Certified Professional Success Coach, Best Selling Author, Motivational Speaker and Success Principles Trainer. Christine has had a successful corporate career, as well as her own business ventures, but Christine's biggest passion lies in helping women reclaim their true identity, find their life purpose, and create a beautiful life, founded on her Relationship Formula—because the most important thing in life is our relationships—with self, higher power, family and friends. This is where Christine truly shines.

Christine has an extensive tool belt. She has worked with legends such as Jack Canfield and John Maxwell and has been employed by Franklin Covey. She is a firm believer in personal development as a part of her self-care routine. Life is all about progress, not perfection.

Christine has been married to her husband, Clawson, for over 23 years. She has 5 sons, 1 daughter-in-law, 2 grandsons, 3 grand-daughters and 2 grand-dogs to date. She loves to dance and dances as often as she can, especially enjoying the opportunities to dance with her high school alumni drill team.

To find out more about hiring Christine to speak at your event or to learn more about her coaching, visit her website at www.christinelavulo.com or find her on LinkedIn, Facebook or Instagram. She would love to connect with you!

FINDING FORREST
Book Excerpt from *Finding Forrest*

Forrest Willett

The Day My Whole World Stopped . . .

October 6, 2002, I lost the most important person in my life in a horrific car wreck. It was not my wife or my son . . . I lost myself.

Yes, I am the man who lost himself. I lost who I was as a husband, father, fireman and friend. I lost my ability to read, write and speak fluently. I was a two year-old child in a 31-year-old body; everything around me was new and extremely frustrating. I could not even control my balance while walking. I looked like a baby deer on a frozen pond trying to stand up straight. Early on, this would cause me to fall down a flight of stairs, breaking my leg and landing me in a wheelchair once again. I often wondered what went wrong, why did this happen? Just weeks before the accident, I was a successful entrepreneur with offices in eight cities and 23 employees. Now I couldn't even count the change to buy a coffee.

At the time of the accident I had my car for sale and a gentleman wanted to take it for a test drive. I handed him the keys and sat in the passenger seat. That's all I remember. Later, through the police investigation, it was revealed that the driver was speaking on his cell phone with his son and lost control of the vehicle at a high rate of speed. The accident scene was one of confusion because even though the car came back as registered to myself, the police and members of the fire department knew that it was not me driving the car. I was a volunteer fire-fighter for 10 years and personally knew everyone in that department. They knew I did not have a moustache or glasses and the person in the passenger seat was unrecognizably swollen, bloody and unconscious with no identification.

My left arm was flopping around and broken in several places. I can't believe how devastated they must have been to see me in this unrecognizable condition. For the previous ten years I was one of the people extracting patients from motor vehicle crashes, now I was the one who needed help. Even my good friend who was a paramedic at the scene later said he could not believe it was me. Yet just hours before I had been at the fire captain's house visiting with my son and feeling on top of the world.

My first memories were 10 days later waking up in the hospital. They were very foggy memories as I slipped in and out of consciousness. The only thing that felt familiar was the constant ringing in my ears and the sound of the blood pressure monitors "beep, beep, beep". My first thought was, "What happened to my arm?" because I could not move it, and "Why is my mouth full of stitches inside and out?" My wife Julie walked into the hospital room with my then two-year-old Hunter. Although I recognized them, I was frustrated that I didn't remember their names. As a matter of fact I didn't remember the names of many people in my life. If you have ever known anyone with Alzheimer's disease or dementia, then you know that losing your memory is one of the most devastating things in life and here I was 31 years old and mine was gone.

All it took was one split second and my life was changed forever. I was left with a traumatic brain injury. Through later testing with the Glasgow Outcome Scale, I was declared to have a catastrophic brain injury. The results stated that I had a permanent loss of 55 percent or more of myself, both mentally and emotionally.

How lucky can one person be? Very few people are given a second chance in life, and I was grateful to be given a third chance. Yes a third, you see this was my second traumatic brain injury. The first occurred when I was two years old and fell down the basement stairs and suffered a subdural hematoma, which required surgical intervention to relieve the pressure from my brain. I have been reminded of this injury and how lucky I am everyday as I wash my hair and run my hand over the area where the bone was removed to relieve the pressure of my swollen brain.

Everything in life had changed. Friends would drop by to visit and tell Julie and I about their weekend of boating at the cottage. When they asked what we had been up to, Julie would share the events of our week, "Forrest learned to brush his teeth and shave on his own and he did not cut his face once. I am so proud of him. And next week he will be working with his speech therapist on a grocery list and if he's feeling up to it he may actually go to the grocery store and try to complete the list with his occupational therapist if his anxiety does not stop him at the door." As friends and visitors would come to the house, they could not help but notice large laminated signs on the refrigerator, stove and doors. They were reminders for me not to touch the stove, to remember to put things back into the refrigerator and to contact someone before I went outside. We also had another person in the house, a rehabilitation support worker, who I called my "babysitter". On the advice of my support team, I needed to have 24-hour attentive care to keep me safe from my own actions. Many people have experienced the frustration of coming out of the mall and forgetting where they've parked their car. I would walk just a few blocks from home and forget where my house was. We were very fortunate to live in a small community where everyone knew each other so when I lost my sense of direction our neighbors would kindly help me get back home. This must have been unbelievably difficult for Julie and I don't know why she stayed with me, but I am grateful that she did. She herself has transformed from a go-getter to a go-giver.

I had a whole team of professionals working with me daily. Some of them were neurologists, psychologists, psychiatrists, surgeons, physiotherapists, speech language pathologists, occupational therapists and the list goes on and on. Close your eyes for a minute and just imagine if you had a dozen or more of the top professionals in their field whose full-time job was to help you get from where you are to where you want to be. Even though they are working with you tirelessly day after day, year after year, the progress is incredibly slow and unfortunately you are not reaching your ultimate goal in the time you wanted. How would you feel?

I began to spiral faster and faster into a deep pit of depression. Anger and despair and the feeling of hopelessness and helplessness became the flavor of the day. My favorite activity became lying in bed all day in between my therapy sessions. I also became dependent on prescription medications, antidepressant-pills, sleeping pills, painkillers such as OxyContin and antidepressants after 14 different surgeries to rebuild my face, arms, hip and leg. At the time, I didn't realize how habit forming the pain relievers would become, just to get through the day. Years later, I now see that the pain relieving effects of these drugs also soothed the pain of a broken heart and broken dreams. Not being able to see a better future can get people hooked on these drugs by chemically removing all of their fear and anxiety.

This was the letter written by my family doctor to the treatment team one and a half years post-accident.

I have known Mr. Willet for over 20 years and I have watched him grow from a young boy into a very successful business person. As you know, he had a major motor vehicle accident on October 6, 2002 at which time Mr. Willett was a passenger in the car that was involved in a single vehicle rollover. He suffered a major traumatic brain injury at the time and was unconscious at the scene, had facial trauma that knocked out several teeth and fractured his left humerus. At the present time, he presents as a pleasant handsome gentleman who is able to carry on a superficial conversation. However, I have major concerns regarding Mr. Willett and that he has trouble with his attention span and cannot hold onto thoughts for a sustained period of time. He has certainly lost a substantial part of his judgement and his ability to speak fluently has been substantially reduced from what it was.

My understanding of the notes from the speech and language pathology assessment is that he has major problems with reading, comprehension and short-term verbal memory. This is well documented in the literature. This gentleman, certainly at present, is unable to function in his job as an entrepreneur at the head of a fairly large and complex company. He certainly does not show the wit and depth of thinking that he had prior to the injury. It is my opinion that he will never be able to go back to the level of work he was doing prior to the injury.

I have concerns that when something like this happens it often leads to breakups in families further down the road and major depression that will further impact on his ability to function as the person he once was.

It is strongly held in my opinion that this gentleman has a psychological and/or mental impairment that will affect his life; at least 55% or more of his ability to function as a father, to make a living and enjoy life, has been changed.— February 12, 2004

A year later, just two and a half years after the date of the accident, a neuropsychological assessment that spanned over four days of testing had concluded that I had plateaued, this means I had reached 95 to 98% of my spontaneous recovery and that I should not expect any further spontaneous recovery.

The doctor said I should feel lucky just to be alive, but I wasn't sure about that. "Two and a half years," that is all they give you? 912.5 days . . . hope has to last longer than that.

This news was another blow to my recovery and diminishing self-esteem. I thought to myself, "How many times can a human being be beaten down and continue to get up?" With all of the diagnoses from the doctors it may look like I was a modern-day Frankenstein. Catastrophic brain injury, clinical depression, several anxiety disorders, post-traumatic stress disorder, mild aphasia and I could go on. I had many thoughts of what's the use, why even try anymore. I could not get excited for the fear of failure was ever looming. I was a real mess. The days and months went up and down between hope, suicidal thoughts and grey numbness in between.

I had no emotions and no control over my own life other than breathing and eating. I felt like a puppet on a string being toted around by well-meaning doctors and therapists. Like a timid little puppy afraid of getting into trouble, I did just as they said, although I felt as If I was getting nowhere.

Everything changed when my favorite hobby of lying in bed finally paid off big-time one morning. I felt as if I had hit the jackpot!

The Day My World Started Again

We all have days in our lives that we will never forget. Something so significant happens that you remember the exact time and place you were, such as the day JFK was shot or the day the twin towers fell in New York on 9/11. You remember where you were, who you were with, and sometimes even what you were wearing.

My significant day came as I was lying in bed with the blankets pulled over my head, waiting for the world to go away. I heard the morning show host on television say, "Coming up next is Jack Canfield with his new book, the Success Principles, how to get from where you are to where you want to be." In my head I thought this is probably more crap, until the commercial was over and they introduced Jack. He claimed that his new book could help anyone get from where they are to where they want to be. He went on to say that your current circumstances and past situations didn't matter. You can transform your life by applying these principles.

For the first time in years, I sat up and pulled the covers off my head. I clearly remember the words Jack said, "If you could do anything in life and there were no limitations, what would you do? I remember chuckling to myself and saying If I could do anything in life and there were no limitations, "I would take my three biggest disabilities and turn them into assets. Not only would I learn to read and write, I would become a #1 best-selling author, and not only would I learn to speak fluently again, I would become a professional speaker and not only would I beat depression and anxiety, I would inspire others to do the same."

Today I am so happy and proud to report that after overcoming many obstacles, starting with gaining the ability to read the Success Principles and applying them to my life on a daily basis; I have accomplished exactly what I set out to do. To say that my life was forever changed and transformed again by applying these principles would be an understatement.

I began by taking 100% responsibility for my life, taking action and a huge desire to get my life back, to experience joy once again, to rebuild what I had lost, to find Forrest again.

Now that I have picked up the pieces and put myself together again with the help of many people, it is my mission to help as many people as I can. It is my trust that you seek your own resources and are relentless in picking up the pieces and putting yourself together once again. If I have been able to do all this with a catastrophic brain injury, severe clinical depression and anxiety, I am positive you can do the same.

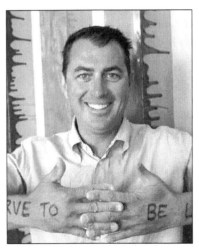

ABOUT FORREST WILLETT

Forrest is a #1 best-selling author and mental health consultant who speaks around the world with individuals and corporations.

Through his keynote speeches and workshops, Forrest promotes mental wellness, helping to decrease days off and sick leave, and to eliminate stigma in the workplace around mental health.

Forrest is also a certified Success Principles trainer and Jack Canfield features his inspirational story in the New York Times Bestseller, *The Success Principles* with over one million books in print.

If you would like to book Forrest to speak, you can connect with him in several ways:

Website: www.mentalhealthspeaker.ca
Facebook: www.facebook.com/profile.php?id=100007210304896
You Tube: *Forrest Willett*

I JUST LIVE

Katherine Williams

Last week I worked on the child/adolescent and adult psychiatric units at a hospital I currently work at in Bismarck, North Dakota. I was able to sit with people who are deep in the trenches of their mental illness. I was able to sit with young people who are feeling afraid, who are feeling vulnerable, who wanted to end their lives before their hospitalization. I got to be someone who instills hope and to utilize therapeutic interventions aimed at reminding them of who they are and that they have an entire life ahead of them. I was able to sit with adults who had been using meth for many years of their lives to the point of hearing auditory hallucinations. I was able to just be present to listen, and to hold a safe space for them to feel comfortable sharing about how they felt as though they will never change. I got to do that. I have a master's degree in social work, I am trained to do this work. My clients and patients trust in my ability to do it. This is my job, but it is much more than that. It is *sacred* to me. This is my calling. This is my purpose and it is a purpose that came out of my own pain.

Today my life is so good. It is a life beyond my wildest dreams, beyond what I ever could have imagined for myself. I am currently a traveling social worker, which means I get paid to do what I love and to travel, which is another love of mine and a coping skill. My housing and meals are paid for. I do my work and I do it well. I show up for myself, my employer, and my patients. I have family and friends who love me and care about me. I have a sponsor. Every night I have a warm bed to sleep in and I actually feel incredibly safe.

It was not always like this.

I had an amazing childhood. I was born into an amazing family. I grew up insanely loved. My parents gave me the world and my grandparents did the same. Even so, growing up, I always knew I was a little different. I remember I would see my peers playing on the playground and yet I was so much more interested in chasing butterflies in the field. I always had a huge imagination and was creative. I would write my own children's books and I loved to draw animals. In my mind I was going to have tons of careers. I would be a meteorologist, an entomologist who specializes in invertebrates, and a brain surgeon. I would play pretend as a mermaid and as the princess of Egypt. The only care in the world I had was trying to figure out how to catch the butterfly or lizard in the yard. I always did though. Little did I know that God had far bigger plans for me which, as I would soon learn, would not come easy.

I was diagnosed with obsessive compulsive disorder (OCD) and major depressive disorder (MDD) when I was 10 years old. I was in 5th grade and hearing my diagnosis felt like a death sentence. I just wanted to be liked. I just wanted to get good grades and I wanted to be "normal." Naturally, I spent a lot of time viewing my life as an unwanted "gift" that I wanted to return to the sender. I had my first suicide attempt two days before I was 11 and I ended up in the child/adolescent unit of a psychiatric unit in the north bay area of California. I spent my 11th birthday there in the hospital and ended up staying a week. I went back twice that same summer with continued suicidal thoughts. I eventually went on to independent study for the remainder of

6th grade. Therapy and going to the psychiatrist were practically my part-time jobs. However, the next battle was about to begin; finding the right medication while in middle school.

A lot of middle school is a blur to me because I spent so much of it under the influence of medications that gave me a range of side effects ranging from intense sedation to feeling extreme emotions to feeling bloated. From the parts I do remember, I remember feeling like I was completely on the outside. I spent hours of my school days in the nurse's office feeling either too depressed to sit upright or too sedated from medication to make it through my classes. I often asked to be picked up to go home because I couldn't stand feeling so sad at school vs. in my own bed. I longed to feel normal and to have normal friendships instead of obsessive friendships where I was so afraid that they would want to distance themselves because I felt like such a loser. I did not know how to articulate any of this to my peers either. I started to identify how I believed others must see me: weird, a loser, not good, not going to amount to anything. I tried over 20 different medications hoping that one day one would work. I felt like a freak, a broken human being who was not even fixable. My mom would watch me cry every day and night. She would hold me and tell me she loved me, "I wish I could wave a magic wand and make it go away." She told me that often. I spent a lot of time at my grandma and papa's house which became my home away from home . . . my safe place. I couldn't imagine ever living life without them.

I had one friend who was with me through all this who is my friend to this day. She was also going through her own pain from mental illness. One time we plotted running away and we were caught doing so. After that, I felt extreme shame and guilt for convincing her to also be a casualty in the war I was battling in my head.

Entering high school meant I was quickly approaching a realm of having to grow up. My high school was much bigger than my middle school and elementary school class combined. Suddenly there were a bunch of new people and new experiences. On my first day of high school I became overwhelmed, ate lunch in the bathroom, and cried on the way home listening to Minnie Driver's music on my iPod. I continued to have an "I hate myself" record player on repeat in my head. College felt like a far-off dream that would never come true. Even so, I managed to find things that bring me some happiness such as theatre where I was able to be someone else and do something I was good at: public speaking and being the center of attention. I had a relationship with God and I attended church and used my gift of singing in choir and in musicals. I also continued to enjoy my childhood hobby, writing. However, my battle with depression and OCD continued to impact my life and the people around me. Regardless of the struggles, I did make a few friends that I have had in my life since those hard times. They have truly seen me through everything.

High school introduced experimentation with men, alcohol, and drugs. I found myself having crushes on boys in high school, yet I felt like I was never the one they wanted. I did receive more male attention though, which was so new to me. I continued to feel like a complete loser and I could not see how anyone would ever like me. One of the ways to numb the pain of what I was experiencing was distracting myself with alcohol and drugs. I was 16 when I had my first drink at a party and immediately I felt . . . good. I felt like I was able to be cool and like I was part of the cool crowd. The following summer I tried marijuana though I was never a fan of that or of smoking. I went to parties with the cool kids as much as I could. I knew the only reason I was "allowed" to go was because of one of my friends. I went to parties in mansions with these people and drank with them, yet I never felt so alone at the same time. I continued to feel like a fish out of water in an incredibly scary pond.

I miraculously graduated from high school and was

accepted to Sacramento State University with a forensic biology concentration. My dream for a while had been to work at a morgue because I had a dream of being a forensic pathologist and it seemed like it actually might become a reality. College surprised me because I actually thrived being away from home. Independence was good for me. I learned how to take care of myself, take my medications without being reminded, and to learn that I was the one responsible for my own mental health. I actually felt like I blended in as a "normal" college student.

My sophomore year of college I started interning at the Sacramento County Morgue and I loved it. I was able to help with the autopsies on a variety of cases including suicides. I could not help thinking to myself how the person in front of me could have been me all those years ago and that now my life was actually . . . getting good. Eventually, I ended up changing concentrations to psychology which was something I was actually good at. I found that the classes that were hard for others (i.e. abnormal psychology, psychopharmacology) were actually very easy for me.

That year I also met a man who I fell absolutely in love with. I always dreamt of this day. After all the fantasy tales I'd read as a young girl, I had this idea that if someone fell in love with me then it meant everything was going to be OK and that I was good enough. It turns out that the man was in love with me too. We became each other's first loves. He accepted me, mental illness and all. When others had run away, he told me "I am sorry you had to go through that." I basked in the glow of love. I watched as childhood dreams I never knew I had manifested. I also began opening up and telling my story of mental illness, but also my story of coming to mental health. My old life felt like lightyears away and I was in a good place. I would talk about my past and people would listen. People wanted to hear more too. I began volunteering for community mental health events, applied and was accepted to an internship as a peer health educator on campus, applied and was awarded a community leadership scholarship, and gained mentors to guide me towards a career I would one day love. I got involved with the Stop Stigma Sacramento Speaker's Bureau as a speaker and was on billboards! MY face was on buses. I found that my passion was telling my story and as a result getting to hear that it helped someone else.

I applied for graduate school, something I never thought I would ever say. I was accepted into the master of social work program right out of college at the age of 22 years old. It dawned on me that I was going to make a career out of the pain I went through. My first year of graduate school I spoke in front of the California state capitol in front of thousands of people. I felt brave. I felt liked. I felt successful. I finally felt like I had achieved happiness which was something that was never in my grasp before.

It all came to a screeching halt when the man I loved broke up with me after 4 years in my final year of graduate school. We had just gotten a dog together. We had a future that I had all planned out. I was devastated. I lost my highly desired internship because I fell into a deep depression that left me unable to get out of bed. I cried at my master's pinning ceremony, I cried at my graduation, and I cried out to God every night praying that He would take away my pain. It was by far the hardest time I had experienced in years. I ended up moving back home with my parents in Milpitas and began working. I began to question decisions I had made including deciding to pursue social work.

Part of me felt like it died with that relationship. I felt like I had a void that I couldn't fill with anything . . . men, alcohol, shopping. I still tried to fill it though. I drank more than I had in college the summer after I graduated. I did so much dating. I was single and desperate not to be. I tried to turn every man I met into "the one." It did not matter if they drank too much, were distant, were dating other women . . . as long as I was being given attention, I told myself I was happy. My life in Sacramento felt light years away. I did whatever I could to not have to feel. I started dating a man who introduced me to cocaine, which I had never done in my life. I was addicted to cocaine the minute it entered my body. It took away the bad feelings and replaced them with confidence, feeling content, without a care in the world. Cocaine soon became my only focus. I spent every day thinking about it, and spent thousands of dollars I didn't have on it. I ditched friends who did not do it. I lied to everyone about where I was and what I was doing. I lost jobs over it or would quit before I was fired. I would do a line to get me through my day and at night I did a line to take the edge off. I lived a complete double life.

Before too long I realized I was indeed addicted. Even though I had dedicated my career to mental health, I knew very little about addiction. I was using it every day, multiple times a day. My nose was bloody and raw nightly. I would act impulsive on it and buy furniture because I was under the influence. Eventually I realized I could not stop using and that I was out of control. I started going to treatment and then immediately stopped because I knew I "wasn't like other addicts."

The worst part of my addiction is that my mental health began to deteriorate. One night I did cocaine, drank a couple drinks, and drove home listening to Christian music. When I got home I took a benzodiazepine on top of the drinks and coke. I was aware how deadly the combination was. I felt like I couldn't breathe and begged God to take my life. *I don't think I can stop, I said* to God that night, praying he would take my addiction away. The next day I was admitted to an inpatient psychiatric unit. I was withdrawing at the hospital. I kicked, screamed, threw things and let out tons of anger that had built up over the years. I convinced them I didn't need to be in the hospital and took back my suicidal ideation. I got out and picked up immediately.

I had a second suicide attempt a few months later after 48 hours of doing cocaine and not sleeping in nearly 72 hours. I wrote a note and took a bunch of pills and was intent on ending my life. I fell deeply asleep but woke up hours later and felt disappointment that I was still alive. I went to get high again.

The following week I landed myself in rehab in Sacramento of all places. I stayed for 90 days and it changed my entire life. I started to rebuild my life, my confidence, and I started really healing. I decided to stay in Sacramento and I started to learn the meaning of peace, true peace. I ended up moving back to the Bay Area for a man. I did start seeing a therapist there to continue my growth. After many days of *one day at a time*, I celebrated my 9th month of sobriety.

I wish I could say that I remained sober on that try but I did not. However, I have found that recovery from addiction is not a linear process. It goes up and down and sideways and then back on track. It may not be everyone's story but it is mine. I see mental health as very similar. Some days are great, some days are not, but there is always a reason to live. Recovery from mental illness takes work, it takes courage, and it is sometimes really hard. For me, recovery looks like taking medications twice a day (including one that reduces my cravings for cocaine), seeing a therapist weekly, seeing a psychiatrist monthly, and a whole bunch of self-care. Speaking of which, self-care looks different for me these days than it ever has. I used to cope with pain by escaping through men, going out drinking, spending hundreds of dollars shopping, or numbing with cocaine. Now it looks like coming home from work after a day of pouring into others who are on a healing journey and instead pouring into my own life. I get myself dressed. I have fun cooking meals for myself and for others. I take my medications. I watch TV. I write. I do things that relax me, make me smile, and that bring me joy. I am learning that I don't need to be around people all the time and that I can sit with myself and be just fine.

Life has a very mysterious way of working out. I learned from a previous roommate at my sober living house that in the end it is always going to be okay as long as I am alive. I can lose my job . . . I'll be okay, I am not going to die. Someone I care about might pass away . . . I will still be okay. I found out I had a mental illness when I was 10 and even though I wanted to die then, today I do not.

Today I get to work with people who are like me and who have often been through things I can relate to. Listening to them share their story is a precious experience that I do not take for granted. I am able to inspire hope and to accept my clients where they are without judgment because I know how hard it is to be there. I recognize their pain. I know that there is not much separating me from them. It is humbling. Every night I go to bed grateful for my life and the love I have in it. My life is not perfect. My recovery is not perfect either. I don't even think there is such a thing as being "fully recovered." There's just . . . living despite it all. It is living with the faith that even though today is a hard day, tomorrow the sun might rise and I will feel better. I have bad days but I have far more good days than I used to. I am glad I stuck around this world to experience it. Today I have hope. There is more to me than the label of an addict. I am not just a person with a mental illness either. I am a person who inspires others. I am a social worker. I am a daughter. I am a person with dreams and purpose. I am a person with faith. I live with mental illness, but most days I just LIVE.

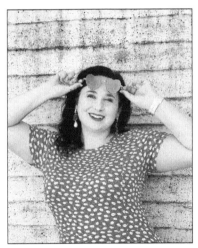

ABOUT KATIE WILLIAMS

Katie's permanent address is in San Jose, California but she is currently located in Bismarck, North Dakota on a traveling social work assignment. You can follow her journey on Instagram @socialworkandsubaru.

Katie holds a master's degree in social work from Sacramento State and is working on obtaining licensure in clinical social work. She is also an advocate for mental health and has told her story at the CA state Capitol, on college campuses, on the radio, and other forms of media. Katie's dream is for mental illness and addiction to be treated equally as physical illness in the workplace. She hopes to one day write a memoir of her own. In her free time Katie enjoys traveling, photography, reading nonfiction, cooking pasta dishes, thrifting, discovering new music, and planning her next adventure in her Subaru Crosstrek. Katie is also the proud dog mom to her corgi Leo.

LIVING BRAVELY AUTHENTIC WITH PTS(D)

Bobbie Jo Yarbrough

This is me daily.
"I don't want to play small."
"I want to help others and create ripples of healing."
"I get so excited about the expansion and helping people live their desires."
This is also me.
"Then why can't I get it started."
"Why can't I just finish this project?"
"Why am I stuck in a space of fear, when rationally I am not fearful?"

All of these thoughts are going through my mind, all at once sometimes. The rational and the seemingly irrational. Me in my excited growth mindset and me feeling trapped in the fixed mindset of my mental illness. Even while I write this, I keep thinking about why there is so much resistance and why do I feel like I have tears in my eyes? Why is it truly so hard to tell my story of growth and healing? Isn't sharing my story exactly what I want to do to inspire growth in others?

And then I realize, the real questions are, "Am I ready to feel all the raw emotions that may come up about being judged? Am I ready to face the stigma placed on my mental health?

Being vulnerable with others can be so scary, however, there is always a part that isn't being shared, like the smaller details. So, in a way, it is still "safe." I can share just enough to connect and relate without giving over too much of myself. Thankfully people don't necessarily need to hear all the trauma details and I don't need to re-traumatize myself by telling them. Being vulnerable with others is scary, but it can seem safer, when you only tell certain things to a smaller group of niched people, in a setting where you have a sense of privacy and like-minded people who support you. Being vulnerable in this way may seem safe, but it's fear-based really and just keeping me playing small. It is keeping me hidden and my mental health stagnates.

I've learned these past few years, being vulnerable with myself is more terrifying. Admitting to myself that I don't have control over the things that are happening to me or what people may think of me, literally makes me feel frozen. Frozen to the point, I feel like I can't breathe, or focus, or even want to be in my "safe" places like my home. I just want to get in the car and drive and drive so I don't have to sit still and feel uncomfortable emotions. I constantly think about moving and relocating to another new city or state where no one knows me. I believe it comes from the space of not having control over the people that have shamed me in the past, silenced my voice, disempowered me, and changed me from the person that I was before. It comes from a space where someone else had the power to change my life and force me to bury all the trauma deep inside me. I silently question whether they will come back and do it again. Most importantly I have learned that I can't be truly vulnerable and courageous and live in this fear.

Being truly vulnerable with myself made me admit that I didn't want to be afraid anymore. I was keeping myself very unsafe and stuck in a trauma loop. I was being retraumatized by my mind. Depression wasn't keeping me safe; it was keeping me in the trauma, reliving the memories, the hurt, the hopelessness. Anxiety and panic attacks were keeping me from answering the door, going out with friends, or picking up groceries. I had become so numb that I couldn't feel the energy and love exchanged when I hugged my kids. Being vulnerable with myself was admitting my children were going to grow up in an unhealthy environment because I was working so hard to be strong and there for the outside world, that my kids were getting my leftovers and I barely had anything left for me to begin with.

I can still remember the day I was sitting in a women's clinic at a VA hospital waiting for my appointment and I looked over and saw a flyer taped to the door, stating if you had experienced MST (Military Sexual Trauma) to call the coordinator listed to connect with their PTSD Team. I remember sitting there just looking at the flyer and feeling a flood of emotions. I was scared, exposed, hopeful, angry, and a longing for someone to help make it all go away. However, I knew at that moment that it was finally time to start the process and to stop hiding. I wanted a healthy intimate relationship. I wanted my kids to have a mom that was whole. I wanted to be whole. So, I took down the number and after a few times of calling and hanging up, I finally left a message. There I did it. Step one is done. Check.

Now here is where I don't want to relive the trauma, and I don't want to gloss over the next few months, of what happened next, because in truth, what happened in the next few months really forced me into a journey of healing, so I will just touch on the pivoting points. After meeting with the VA PTSD Team and promising myself, I would trust the process. The man I was in a relationship with became very volatile and I found myself in a circle of domestic violence. I learned that he also suffered from severe mental illness and was not only refusing to take the medications prescribed, but he was also self-medicating with alcohol. I share this because at one point I was his understanding partner, I was a social worker, I was a fellow veteran, I also experienced trauma. I loved him and his children very much, and he cried and asked me to help him. I was an empath who was helping others with their mental illness every day for my career, who would I be if I didn't help someone that I loved? So of course, I put my healing on hold (without even realizing it), to help hold our families together, while things got worse and worse. I retreated into the safety of hiding my trauma from my friends and hardly anyone knew what was happening.

The major difference this time was that I was a mom now. I couldn't hide this from my daughter. I saw what it was doing to her too and it was breaking my heart. She started therapy, was immediately diagnosed with an anxiety disorder, and carried a stuffed "therapy dog" to school every day, which she was allowed to keep in her cubby. She even started asking me if she could "work from home" with me because she was scared every time she saw a vehicle similar to his.

And there it was. My worst fear as a mom. I couldn't keep us safe. I couldn't keep my child safe. I couldn't protect her from trauma. And then I found out I was pregnant. I can't put into words what it was like for me to experience trauma like this as a mom. It's not just you being affected anymore. My mental health was a mess, my physical body was growing another life while in a trauma state, and I knew that now my choices were passing on generational trauma to two kids that didn't deserve it. So much self-blame. So much guilt. I loved them both so much and I couldn't feel it. I couldn't feel love. I didn't know if I ever would be able to again.

"What kind of mom am I?" "They would be better with someone else." "I should do what is best for them and consider adoption." This was my self-talk. As someone who grew up in the foster care system and had an adult foster daughter currently in college, these were all things I never in my life thought I would say, much less start to believe. But one day I left work early, left a message for my therapist, sobbing, telling her just that. Then at 0530 the very next morning, I was told they had found my friend's body and he had taken his life. He left his amazing wife and three children. He had been battling combat PTSD and TBI for years after serving in the military. That day I realized that I couldn't let this happen to my children. That me leaving them wasn't the answer. That leaving the situation, the city, the trauma was the first change that was needed. I had to change for them. I wanted to change for myself.

I share all of this because this was how real and deep the mental illness was growing inside me, as I kept trying to "handle it on my own by being strong." In reality, all I was doing was burying my truths and burying my trauma deeper and deeper. I needed to empower myself to heal and speak my truth and stop retreating. I needed to find the courage to stand in my power.

One day I woke up and realized I had actually changed my entire life. When I think about it now, I don't think I really knew I was doing it. I was just so determined to live in my truth and stop letting the traumas others were causing me, control me. I just kept asking from my heart and held space for what I wanted my life to be like for myself and my kids. I kept connecting myself with people and programs that were healthy and supportive.

And then, I was introduced to a PTSD support program for Veterans and First Responders called The Battle Within. I remember the fear I had of feeling exposed. Ironically, I was so scared to let go of it all. I was so scared to feel it all again. But I did. I felt it and I released it. And every day since I release a little more. I can explore what living my best life truly means now. I am not the same person I was "before." I had to let her go. I had to tell my ego and protector that we couldn't be truly safe from a space of fear. I had to embody all the parts of me without guilt and shame. It was then that I started to love myself from my heart space.

After my week there, the very first thing I did when I walked through my door was hug all my kids. Really long, love felt hugs. And I asked each of them, "How can momma love you more?" I knew then, that no matter what has happened in the past, my kids truly love me and know I will always keep them safe. Sometimes I just sit silently and feel their love and feel all the emotions of being loved. It is the best.

Within a few months on my life-changing Hero's Journey, I became a Certified Sacred Soul Alignments and Sacred Light Practitioner. Using these powerful alignments, activations, and heart-centered healing modalities to heal me and my traumas. I founded Bravely Authentic, LLC to assist people to connect to their heart space, heal and release trauma, and tap into their clarity. I tell them all the time, "you have a vision of what you want now but it's going to be even better. Keep showing up for yourself and ask from your heart's space." Co-creating life-changing spaces of healing and clarity puts me in such a space of love and gratitude every single day.

"I deserve all the things I want and desire."

"I am loved so, so much."

"I am committed to my growth and healing."

"Ease and grace always."

Yes, I live with PTS(D) and I do it being Bravely Authentic

Bravely Authentic, LLC
Transformational Healing, Intuitive Guidance, and Sacred Support

ABOUT BOBBIE JO

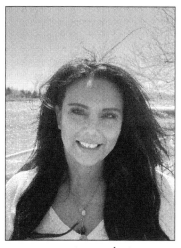

Bobbie is the Founder of Bravely Authentic, LLC. She is a trauma-informed Transformational Healing Practitioner, where she helps her clients take back their control, heal from trauma, and reconnect with their self-love through Transformational Healing, Intuitive Guidance, and Sacred Supports, so they can create the life they truly desire. She uses a combination of energy healing modalities, subconscious reprogramming techniques, and her experiences as a social worker, mentor, and leader to create trauma-informed spaces of growth and healing just for her clients.

Bobbie jo graduated from San Diego State University School of Social Work, after serving six years in the U.S. Navy. She is a graduate of Intuitive Insights: School of Intuition San Diego, Certified Sacred Soul Alignment™ Practitioner (SSAA Candidate 2021), a Sacred Light™ III Practitioner, Reiki Master, and Money Reiki Master, Certified in Neuro-Linguistic Programming (NLP), Emotional Freedom Techniques (EFT), Hypnosis, T.I.M.E. Techniques, FIRES Method, and Life & Success Coaching.

Bobbie jo has over 11 years of assisting both youth and adults with trauma-informed transformations in their day-to-day lives. She understands what it is like to live with PTSD and is continuously on her Hero's Journey to whole health. She strives to create a legacy of self-love for her children and a space of healing for those who want to live in their joy again.

By healing ourselves, we create ripples of healing throughout the world.

ACKNOWLEDGMENTS

FACES OF MENTAL ILLNESS

This book is made possible through the generous financial contributions of Claudia and Samantha. They are both passionate about breaking the stigmas surrounding mental illness and creating a movement towards inclusive mental health. They are dedicated to bringing awareness to the world on this topic, because mental illness is not always what you think. They are both graduates and certified trainers of Jack Canfield Success Principles Training and met in 2019 at one of his events. Immediately upon meeting and discussing their own lives, they felt a huge pull to collaborate in this important and much needed project.

Thank you readers for making our dream a reality

Our special thanks to Jack Canfield for all your teachings, mentoring, and guidance which led us to make this book become a reality, and especially for saying YES to writing the Foreword of our book. This means the world to us.

To Marielle Vaughn-Hickman for the inspiration, you provided for the book's name, to Dr. Deb Sandella, Patty Aubery, and Kathleen Seeley for their kind reviews, to Kate Butler, our publisher who immediately said YES to this project as she knows how important this topic is and how much the world needs to hear these stories and finally, to each one of the brave individuals who said YES to sharing their stories and personal struggle while living with mental illness to bring awareness to the world.

This movement has been sponsored by: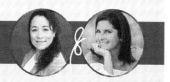

CLAUDIA FERNANDEZ-NIEDZIELSKI

Founder and Co-Creator of the Global "Faces of Mental Illness" Movement, our journey from Stigma to Health, #1 International Best Selling Author, Transformational Speaker, & Entrepreneur.

> *Armed with all these tools and a* **"** *new understanding of what is possible when we put our mind to it and apply these lessons; inspired me to begin a new journey where I can share this message with as many people as I can.*

Claudia's journey began in 2011 when her search for a way out of situations that appeared impossible to overcome, would lead her to cross paths with the Master of Transformation, Jack Canfield.

As a result, she would end up unlocking the secrets to turn her life completely around and create a new path towards happiness! Now she guides others through this process with her personal and business coaching, workshops, and webinars.

HER PHILOSOPHY IS VERY SIMPLE:
Assist clients to FIRST identify who they are, what is holding them back, acknowledge and embrace the positive past, recognize and heal the negative past and guide them to create that strong and solid foundation they will need to honor their goals, their feelings, their dreams and themselves.

grab a copy of my books...

WOMEN WHO RISE and WOMAN WHO ILLUMINATE

These 30 stories will speak to your heart and lift up your soul. Each chapter follows the journey that led each co-author to rise above challenges in their own life. These pages reflect the intimate choices that were made to rise above challenging situations and as a result live extraordinary lives. This is the sixth book in the #1 International Best-selling Inspired Impact Book Series.

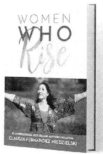

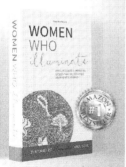

#1 AMAZON BESTSELLER!

WORK WITH CLAUDIA

UNLOCK YOUR GOLDEN ESSENCE
YOUR INNER POWER

Excellent opportunity for business owners, individuals, students, and staff who are interested in learning the tools necessary to:

- Process the past and leave it behind
- Select the best influences in your life
- Participate in life in a way that creates miracles
- Feel alive, excited, and full of joy
- Increase your confidence

UNLOCK THE SECRETS TO YOUR PEAK PERFORMANCE

This workshop will provide you with all the tools necessary to propel your life to the next level.

Learn how to:

- Take charge of your life
- Spark the fire in your life so you can ignite your FUTURE
- Create the life you always wanted
- Improve your results
- Increase your income
- and so much more

KEYNOTE SPEAKING/TRANSFORMATIONAL

If you are looking for someone to inspire transformation with your audience through a story of adversity and obstacles to one of triumph and success, look no further.

Claudia is poised to create an atmosphere of trust, love, and compassion for anyone in the audience as she shares her very own story of resilience and the tools and principles she has used to transform and create a life with purpose and joy despite her mental illness diagnosis at the early age of 22; the devastating chronic illness of her husband and young daughter, and the abandonment her son felt during these years.

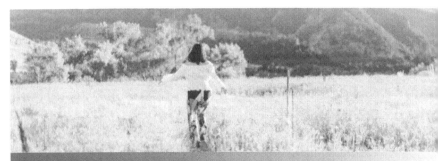

GOING THROUGH CHANGE CAN BE TOUGH
doing it alone can be tougher.

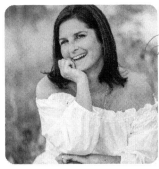

Hello! I'm Samantha.
Please call me Sam.

My mission is to change the way the world views mental health, so people can openly speak about whatever issues they have and get the help they not only need but deserve without fear of judgment, labels, and repercussions.

GRIEF IS A VERY PERSONAL JOURNEY.
BUT YOU DON'T HAVE TO GO THROUGH IT ALONE.

Introducing...

griefhab™ *Get unlimited access to me!*

There's no other program like this.
Griefhab eliminates the waiting, the waiting rooms, the therapists agenda.

THIS IS ABOUT GRIEVING YOUR WAY!

Visit **www.samantharuth.com** to learn more

The
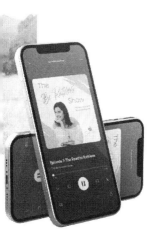

Be Ruthless
Show

Making Noise and
Breaking Stigmas

Listen to my podcast.

A place where we'll be having the conversations other people don't. The conversations other people won't.

Because. Mental. Health. Matters.

 Spotify Listen on
Apple Podcasts

ALSO CHECK OUT

Ruthless Merchandise

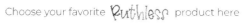

Together let's raise awareness by wearing your soft and cozy "Ruthless" hoodie, shirt or hat, and other souvenir items you will love to have.

Choose your favorite *Ruthless* product here

www.samantharuth.com/shop

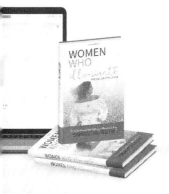

Also, grab a copy of Women Who Illuminate. Featuring a collection of 30 illuminating stories to inspire your soul's journey.

We also dive deeper into my story of self-discovery, pain, loss, healing, persistence, and ultimately learning to accept and embrace my TRUE self.

I hope this will help you see your quirks as your strengths and give you the inspiration to turn your pain into power.

GRAB A COPY OF THE BOOK HERE
www.samantharuth.com/shop

BECOME A SPONSOR

FACES OF MENTAL ILLNESS
20 STORIES bringing you through the journey from stigma to health

Join our movement!

BECOME A SPONSOR
FOR THE NEXT BOOK

REACH OUT TO:

Samantha Ruth

📞 +1 (248) 730 5544

✉ sam@samantharuth.com

Claudia Fernandez-Niedzielski

📞 (916) 248-3004 Direct

✉ ClaudiaImpactsLives@gmail.com

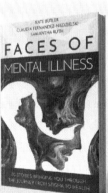

RESOURCES:

SUGGESTED READING AND
ADDITIONAL RESOURCES FOR HEALING

1. The 30 day sobriety solution – (Alcohol addiction) Jack Canfield and Dave Andrews

2. The Success Principles, How to get from where you are to where you want to be – Jack Canfield

3. Goodbye hurt and pain – (Emotional intelligence book for a life of success) – Dr. Deborah Sandella

4. An unquiet mind (Life with manic depressive disorder) – Dr. Kay Redfield Jaminson

5. Touched by Fire – (History of mental illness in all creative souls) – Dr. Kay Redfield Jaminson

6. Healing the hardware of your soul – (Healing tips for all those with a mental illness) – Dr. Daniel Amen

7. Change your brain, change your life (How to conquer many mental illnesses) – Dr Daniel Amen

8. Your brain is always listening – (Tame the dragons that control our happiness) – Dr. Daniel Amen

9. The end of Mental Illness – (Neuroscience and mental illness) Dr. Daniel Amen

10. Healing ADD – (How to heal the 7 types of ADD) – Dr. Daniel Amen

11. Finding Forrest – (A journey of recovery after a terrible accident) – Forrest Willett

12. Shattered Together – (How to navigate life and heal after the suicide of a love one) – Cathleen Elle

13. In Sickness and in Mental Health (How a married couple with mental illness can survive) – Diane Mitz

14. Breakdown – (A clinician's experience in a broken system of emergency psychiatry) – Lynn Nanos LICSW.

15. A Woman's Worth – Marianne Williamson

16. The Fruitful Darkness – (A journey through Buddhist Practice and tribal wisdom) – Joan Halifax

17. Second Sight – (How to discover your intuitive gifts) – Judith Orloff

18. Spiritual Emergence – (When personal transformation becomes a crisis) – Stanislav Grof and Christina Grof,

19. Emergence (The shift from ego to essence) – Barbara Marx Hubbard

20. 52 Codes for Conscious Self Evolution – (A process of metamorphism to realize our full potential self)- Barbara Marx Hubbard

21. I am Not Sick I Don't Need Help (How to help someone with a mental illness accept treatment) – Xavier Amador

22. The book of hope (101 voices on overcoming adversity) – Jonny Benjamin

23. Man's search for meaning – Viktor Frankl

24. Mortal Engines (fiction) – Philip Reeve

25. Self Love (workbook for women) – Megan Logan MSW, LICSW

26. The Dialectical Behavior Therapy Skills Workbook – Practical DBT Exercises for Learning Mindfulness, Interpersonal Effectiveness, Emotions Regulation and Distress Tolerance) – Matthew McKay, Jeffrey C. Wood and Jeffrey Brantley

27. It didn't start with you (How inherited family trauma shapes who we are and how to end the cycle) – Mark Wolynn

28. A First-Rate Madness (Uncovering the links between Leadership and Mental Illness) – Nassir Ghaemi

29. The Battle Within – PTSD support program for Veterans and First Responders

Helpful Websites

Stopstigmasacramento.org
Nami.org
MentalHealth.gov
Erasethestigmanow.org
Reachouttogether.com
mentalhealthfirstaid.org
psychcentral.com
headtohealth.gov.au
verywellmind.com
calmsage.com
7cups.com (free 24/7 chat)
happiful.com
themighty.com
doxy.me

For the most visited mental health sites visit:
psychreg.org/most-visited-mental-health-websites

REPRINTED WITH PERMISSIONS

Jack Canfield
Claudia Fernandez-Niedzielski
Samantha Ruth
Kate Butler
Samantha Dee Niedzielski
Sarah Abbott
Laura Asay-Bemis
Rebecca Bakken
David Bartley
Natalie Conrad
Joanna Dorman-Blackstock
Cathleen Elle
Henry Johnstone
Tad Lusk
Loraine Marshall
Diane Mintz
Mehreen Siddiqui
Susan Sims Hillbrand
Christine Whitehead Lavulo
Forrest Willett
Katherine Williams
Bobbie Jo Yarbrough

REVIEWS

"Fernandez-Niedzielski, Ruth and Butler with their new book *Faces of Mental Illness* have cracked open the stigma of mental illness to reveal real people with touching human stories; their lives demonstrate how resilience and courage can navigate a journey to health. It's time we see human faces instead of diagnoses behind what we label Mental Health. Our community of humankind is diverse and each person's journey unique. Mental illness is part of that journey for some the same way diabetes if for others. This book will open your heart and dissolve artificial separations amongst us. I recommend it."

—Deborah Sandella PhD, RN, #1 International Bestselling author of *Goodbye Hurt & Pain, 7 Simple Steps to Health, Love and Success*, and Creator of RIM, a heavily-backed neuroscience tool proven to reduce stress and improve quality of life. As seen in CNN, CBS, NBC, FOX and USA Today.

"*Faces of Mental Illness* is a book that grabs your attention immediately as you are fully immersed in the lives of these 20 brave individuals who have experienced such a wide range of mental illness symptoms and circumstances that most of us could not even begin to imagine; and yet, they have all found a way to live productive and positive lives. The real, raw and authentic stories you will find in this book paint the perfect picture of what is possible despite Mental Illness and invite us to join the movement to stop the stigma on an illness that is widely spread and highly misunderstood. I have certainly gained so much more compassion and understanding for these individuals as I have come to know several of them personally and would have never imagined they were struggling with mental illness. I highly recommend this book."

—Kathleen Seeley, Founder: Massively Human Leadership

This is more than just a book. *Faces of Mental Illness* is a movement, created by two women with a mission to break the stigmas surrounding mental illness and who are being supported by a publisher who wholeheartedly believes in this message. What Fernandez-Niedzielski, Ruth and Butler have created will move you, will inspire you; and most importantly, will give you hope. In this world full of stigmas, these 20 brave individuals will open your eyes to what it's truly like to live with a mental illness and still thrive! A must read!"

—Patty Aubery, Co-Creator of the billion-dollar publishing brand, "Chicken Soup for the Soul®", President of The Canfield Training Group, and #1 Best-Selling Author of *Permission Granted*

Made in the USA
Las Vegas, NV
08 December 2021

36570524R00101